DISEASE, DIAGNOSES, AND DOLLARS

DISEASE, DIAGNOSES, *and* DOLLARS

Facing the Ever-Expanding Market for Medical Care

Robert M. Kaplan

C

COPERNICUS BOOKS
An Imprint of Springer Science+Business Media

© 2009 Springer Science+Business Media, LLC

Published in the United States by Copernicus Books,
an imprint of Springer Science+Business Media.

Copernicus Books
Springer Science+Business Media
233 Spring Street
New York, NY 10013
www.springer.com

Library of Congress Control Number:
2008935538

Manufactured in the United States of America.
Printed on acid-free paper.

ISBN 978-0-387-74044-7   e-ISBN 978-0-387-74045-4

Preface

Good health is our most precious asset. Without health, life becomes much more challenging. Because health is so central in our lives, we invest trillions of dollars to achieve more wellness or to remedy diseases. A vast healthcare establishment is ready and willing to receive these investments. Some investments in healthcare result in healthier and happier citizens. Other investments have little effect on health, are wasteful, and even harmful.

It is widely acknowledged that there is a serious crisis in American healthcare. There is no real healthcare system in the USA. Instead, we have a patchwork of competing systems. Medicare covers the elderly and people with some defined problems, such as kidney failure. Medicaid covers the blind, the disabled, and families with dependent children. Most people have private insurance that is paid for by their employers. The public systems are in financial trouble, and an increasing number of employers claim that they are no longer able to pay for insurance. The number of uninsured or underinsured people in the USA has soared to well over 45 million.

Proposals for national health insurance abound. However, virtually all of the proposals focus on providing coverage for all people. Although universal healthcare is an attractive goal, there is another problem. We have been persuaded to want more healthcare than we need. A *New York Times* article by columnist by Gena Kolata [1] described patients lining up for all of the care that Medicare will cover. The article describes patients in a Florida clinic seeking every service that the Medicare program will pay for. They ask for the latest diagnostic tests, and they want the latest medicines that they have learned about by watching advertisements on television. The Medicare system, in some ways, encourages this. If a service is covered, the provider only needs to send in the bill and he will be paid. Is all of this medical care necessary?

This book is about some disquieting conflicts between consumers and their healthcare providers. Our healthcare system is big and complicated: it is the largest sector in the biggest economy in the history of the world. But, unlike other industries, healthcare has not been held accountable for what it produces. We know, for example, that the USA spends significantly more per capita on healthcare than any other country. Yet, we rank last among comparison countries in the Organization for Economic Cooperation and Development on the major health indicators. We also know that there are substantial regional differences in healthcare expenditures within the USA. Even when we adjust for a variety of variables, such as age distribution, poverty, education, or minority status, regions that spend more do not have better outcomes, and some evidence suggests that quality of care is lower in the regions that spend more, not less, on healthcare.

Our problem is not that providers charge too much, it is that they do too much. We assume that the high costs of healthcare reflect the expense of services and medications. *Disease, Diagnosis, and Dollars* calls this assumption into question. Drug prices in the USA are not significantly higher in comparison with that in other developed countries, because few patients actually pay the listed retail price. Total costs are a function of two factors: unit price and volume. Volume, not unit cost, may be driving our healthcare crisis. The following chapters suggest that mass markets have been created for services that may offer little or no benefit to patients. Many of these markets are for preventive medicine. These include cancer-screening tests, and medications to control blood pressure, cholesterol, and glucose. The attractiveness of preventive medicine is that it can make well people a market for expensive pharmaceutical products and tests.

These mass markets have been nurtured with the support of respected panels of experts who have created guidelines for new tests to diagnose illness and new drugs to treat disease. New revisions of these guidelines are unlikely to benefit most consumers of healthcare. Still, these guidelines are used to set standards for the practice of medicine, and quality of care is often defined as adherence to the standards. Once the guidelines are set, doctors follow them. We have been intentionally led to believe tests and medicines will offer greater benefits than evidence supports. The result: uncontrollable costs and minimal benefits.

There are consequences to the overuse of medications and tests. Although most screening tests and modern medicines used in prevention are safe for individuals, their use runs up the costs of healthcare. High costs result in higher insurance premiums for all of us. As more employers drop health insurance for their employees when costs accelerate, the expanded use of ineffective preventive medicine may have the unintended consequence of increasing the number of uninsured patients, potentially damaging the health of others in the community.

The concluding chapters offer suggestions for policy makers and for patients. Methods for systematically evaluating the cost-effectiveness of new guidelines are discussed. The final chapter provides practical suggestions to enable patients to share in decisions about treatments or tests that can have uncertain benefits.

Many colleagues have contributed to the development of this manuscript. I started thinking about these problems 10 years ago during a sabbatical year at the Dartmouth Medical School. That year I got to know Elliott Fisher, Gil Welch, Lisa Schwartz, and Jack Wennberg. The Dartmouth experience shaped my thinking about overuse in medical care. The ideas for the book have been shaped by a dozen years of experience as a faculty member for the American Health Association US Seminar on the Epidemiology and Prevention of Cardiovascular Disease. The core of the book has been adapted from the lectures I offered at the Lake Tahoe seminar. While a professor at the University of California, San Diego School of Medicine, close colleagues including Rick Kronick, Robert Langer, and Ted Ganiats discussed these ideas with me on many occasions. I am particularly indebted to Mike Criqui, a noted physician epidemiologist who, over the course of 25 years, systematically taught me the basics of epidemiology and helped sharpen my thinking. Mike may not agree with all of the ideas in this book, but I hope he will see that he inspired some of the critical reflection. At UCLA, I benefited from feedback from Gerald Kominski, Tom Rice, Bill Cononar, Dominick Frosch, and several others. Readings of early chapters by Andrea Grefe and Margaret Gaston guided the direction and the prose. I am most sincerely appreciative for the detailed feedback I received from Paul Farrell from Springer and Copernicus Press. Paul critiqued every page, challenged the thinking and the writing, and made the manuscript better in countless ways. My senior editor Bill Tucker has also been exceptionally helpful. Finally, I am most indebted to the Rockefeller Foundation who provided a quiet study in Bellagio overlooking Lake Como Italy, where the manuscript was finally completed. The fellow resident scholars at Bellagio also provided very valuable feedback.

I expect that many intelligent and well-informed readers will disagree with some of the basic premises in these chapters: the book was intended to be provocative. However, the text is built upon data from contemporary, peer-reviewed literatures in medicine and health services research. I hope the book stimulates debate, fosters new research, and makes us wiser consumers of healthcare.

Robert M. Kaplan
rmkaplan@ucla.edu
Los Angeles, California
June 2007

Reference

1. Kolata G. Patients in Florida lining up for all that Medicare covers. *New York Times*, 2003.

Contents

List of Figures

List of Tables

Chapter 1
Disease, Outcomes, and Money

I can still remember the call. At age 77, Sally, a close friend of the family, had a positive mammogram. I was a professor at the medical school, and her family wanted to know the names of the best breast surgeon and the most distinguished medical oncologist. We all want the best medical interventionists when faced with a potentially fatal illness. After a biopsy, Sally learned that she had a condition called ductal carcinoma in situ, or DCIS. The doctors told Sally that this was a mild form of breast cancer, but the family was unwilling to take chances. She got surgery, chemotherapy, and radiation therapy. Today, Sally is alive and doing well.

After treatment, family members became advocates for early detection in older women. They believed that Sally's life had been saved because her doctor was "aggressive." He ordered a mammogram and followed up the positive result with a biopsy, surgery, chemotherapy, and radiation. How can anyone argue with his judgment?

The problem is that Sally suffered considerably. The suffering began with severe anxiety and fear of death. Then surgery, chemotherapy, and radiation therapy took a heavy toll: She lost her hair, lost her energy, and even considered whether death might be a better alternative than continuing medical torture. The aftermath of the treatment included continuing anxiety, concern about memory loss, and depression. New evidence suggests that younger women who receive chemotherapy are much more likely to have serious adverse side effects than was previously recognized. As many as 61 percent of younger privately insured women with breast cancer require hospitalization or visit emergency rooms for serious adverse consequences of their treatment [1]. So, in terms of the pain and suffering caused by the so-called "side effects," Sally paid dearly for her treatment. And what is more, it is uncertain that the treatment had a significant impact on how long Sally lived. In many countries, screening mammography is not done for women of Sally's age, and the chances of death from breast cancer in these counties are about the same as they are in the USA [2]. Ductal breast cancer is common in women over 65, and the best evidence suggests that without diagnosis and treatment, the majority of them continue their lives and die of other causes without ever knowing they had cancer [3].

R.M. Kaplan, *Disease, Diagnoses, and Dollars*, DOI 10.1007/978-0-387-74045-4_1,   1
© Springer Science+Business Media, LLC 2009

For anyone who has thought seriously about health and healthcare, Sally's case—statistically "typical," a perfectly "ordinary" case—the questions raised are anything but ordinary. In addition to the undeniable physical and emotional consequences of her diagnosis and treatment, the interventions were costly, and these costs accrued not only to Sally and her family. Sally was a Medicare patient and paid only a portion of her own medical expenses. However, Medicare costs are out of control, and each time the costs go up there is pressure to cut expenses elsewhere [4], in the hospital, in the healthcare system, and in society at large. Anyone's individual journey through serious illness and treatment is by its very nature a tremendous personal challenge. But there is another urgent challenge we face together as a society, and how we address it could have huge consequences for the health of the population.

Buying Health, Buying Healthcare

This book is about using our healthcare resources to buy the most health for the most people. Buying health and buying healthcare are not equivalent. We face a paradox of excess and deprivation. Some people get too much healthcare, including expensive but ineffective tests and treatments. Experts believe that between one-third and one-half of all of the services purchased and delivered by our healthcare system have no beneficial effect on patients [5].

The overuse of services has negative consequences for at least two reasons. First, excessive use forces the costs of healthcare to increase. In the US healthcare system, increased costs are passed on to employers, who pay most of the health insurance costs. As costs increase, many employers decide to discontinue coverage for their employees. The result is that the uninsured rate increases [6, 7]. Today, nearly 50 million US citizens are without health insurance [8]. In a kind of paradox, excess and deprivation are causally linked. Over-consumption causes insurance rates to rise, resulting in an increase in deprivation for the most vulnerable portion of the population.

The second reason excessive use is a concern in that exposure to medical care is not without risk. A report from the Institute of Medicine of the National Academies of Science suggests that complications of medical care are the third leading cause of death in the USA [9, 10]. Even though screening tests such as mammography seem very safe, there may be consequences. The United States Preventive Services Task Force does not recommend mammography for women before age 50 [11]. There is no evidence from major clinical trials to suggest that screening mammography before menopause leads to an extension of life expectancy [12, 13]. However, among women who begin mammography in their late thirties, as recommended by some professional societies, the chances are 1 in 3 that they will have a false-positive result by age 50 [14]. These false positives lead to painful and anxiety-provoking biopsies and can be quite threatening. There is considerable fear, anxiety, pain, and expense. Patient benefit is often minimal, and harm can be a reality.

Is More Better?

My personal attachment to the problems has come through an unusual course. I am a Ph.D. rather than an M.D. So, I approach the problem from a different angle than a practicing physician. However, I have a great deal of familiarity and empathy for the challenges facing medical practitioners. As a professor in a School of Public Health, I study health policy. I came to this position after more than 30 years as a professor in a medical school. During those years, I participated in nearly all of the courses in the medical school and the programs for training primary care physicians. The last 8 of the 30 years were spent as chair of a Department of Family and Preventive Medicine. Among other tasks, I had responsibility for the oversight of a substantial medical practice in an era when managed care became dominant in the medial landscape. Patients complained that they did not get all of the services they wanted, and frustration with managed-care companies became rampant. Why don't those cheap companies get in line and pay for the services their insured patients deserve? Believe me, as a patient and a family advocate for other patients, I shared these frustrations.

An easy solution to our problems in healthcare is to recognize that healthcare is important and that we need to spend money for good service. Every medical specialty group lobbies for more coverage. We need more money for primary care, more money for specialty care, more money for the care of children, more money for the care of the elderly, and more money for the care of disenfranchised groups. In addition, we need more money for research, more money for allied health professionals, more money for community health centers. . . .

But will more money heal the problem? The US healthcare system is the most expensive sector in the biggest economy in the history of the world. On a per capita basis, nobody approaches our expenditures. The UK spends only about $0.40 for each dollar spent in the USA, and more or less the same story holds in other developed countries: Belgium and Denmark spend only about $0.50 for each dollar spent in the USA, and Spain spends only about $0.33 [15].

What is our extra expenditure purchasing? One of the most important unexplored assumptions in healthcare policy is that greater expenditure will result in better health. We know from international studies that developed countries that spend considerably less on healthcare have about equal health outcomes. The health of nations is typically compared using measures of life expectancy or infant mortality. Even though the UK spends well less than half of what the USA spends per capita, life expectancy in the UK is slightly greater than it is in the USA, and infant mortality rates are slightly lower. Among thirteen countries in one recent comparison, the USA ranked twelfth when compared on sixteen health indicators [16].

Within the USA, there is considerable variability in healthcare spending. For example, using data from the Medicare program, the per capita spending ranges from a low of $2,736 in Oregon to a high of $6,307 in Alaska. State-level data are also available on the average quality of healthcare. Quality is typically defined as adherence to defined standards of patient care. For example, it is possible to estimate the extent to which physicians adhere to defined patient guidelines. There appears to be little association between per capita spending and the quality of care patients receive [17]. Spending more does not buy better quality of care. In fact, states that spend more per Medicare recipient appear to have lower quality care. In medical practice, specialists are more expensive than primary care doctors. The states that spend the most are those with a higher percentage of medical specialists and fewer primary care doctors [17]. Some analyses show that areas that have more primary care doctors, not more specialists, have better health outcomes. Adjusting for socioeconomic status does not alter this finding.

What Is Wrong?

Fixing problems in healthcare may sound easy. Hundreds, if not thousands, of politicians, policy experts, government officials, academics, healthcare professionals, and even authors have offered solutions. However, despite the application of the very best minds and the expenditure of an ungodly amount of money, we have made remarkably little progress in the quest to fix American healthcare. A major premise of this book is that we have failed because we have been guided by some basic beliefs and these beliefs may be incorrect.

In the following chapters some basic notions will be examined. Some of the questions to be considered include:

Will improved diagnostic technology result in better population health?
Must all disease be eradicated?
Is more healthcare always better?
Should we promote public-health screening for diseases such as cancer and heart disease?
Is early detection the best approach to preventive medicine?

With some qualifications, this book takes a controversial position: The answer to each of these questions is "no." The justification for these conclusions is explained in the next few chapters. To set the stage, though, a conceptual model is offered first. The model challenges the belief that modern medicine is well equipped to eradicate chronic diseases such as cancer and heart disease. We have failed to recognize that most important chronic diseases evolve over decades in a person's body. By the time they come to medical attention, they are well-entrenched and not subject to cure. Treatment may alleviate some of the suffering from these conditions, but care may also cause problems that harm our overall level of well being.

Few of us will escape chronic illnesses, but the good news is that our lives may be unaffected by some of these conditions. In fact, we might be better off not knowing about some of the disease that is already established within our bodies. And looking for these problems may not be a fruitful exercise. Some diagnoses lead to unnecessary treatment. Furthermore, aggressive programs to find new disease might have other public-health consequences. When we use public-health resources for one purpose, we give up the opportunity to spend money that could have achieved better outcomes for another problem. This problem will be considered later in this book. Finally, the implications of the model for public health and its relationship to actual medical decisions will be explored. In the final chapter, I offer methods for patients to become better consumers of their own healthcare.

In summary, the goal of this book is to offer a different way of thinking about problems in healthcare and preventive medicine. A few disclaimers are necessary. Many intelligent and well-informed people will disagree with some or even all of the basic premises. That is expected. If the book is not provocative, I will not have achieved one of my primary goals: to provoke thought and positive change. Second, I can say with certainty that these ideas warrant additional research. Scientifically conclusive tests are not currently available for many of my assertions. However, the evidence supporting the concepts is quite substantial. Wherever possible, I support my assertions with the best contemporary research evidence I can find. And finally, I do hope that the ideas offer enough challenge to open new and different conversations about and explorations of healthcare and preventive medicine policy.

References

1. Hassett MJ, O'Malley AJ, Pakes JR, Newhouse JP, Earle CC. Frequency and cost of chemotherapy-related serious adverse effects in a population sample of women with breast cancer. *J Natl Cancer Inst.* Aug 16 2006;98(16):1108–1117.
2. Shapiro S, Coleman EA, Broeders M, et al. Breast cancer screening programmes in 22 countries: current policies, administration and guidelines. International Breast Cancer Screening Network (IBSN) and the European Network of Pilot Projects for Breast Cancer Screening. *Int J Epidemiol.* Oct 1998;27(5):735–742.
3. Welch HG. *Should I Be Tested for Cancer?* Berkeley, CA: University of California Press; 2004.
4. Gilmer T, Kronick R. It's the premiums, stupid: projections of the uninsured through 2013. *Health Aff (Millwood).* Apr 5 2005.
5. Relman AS. Shattuck Lecture–the health care industry: where is it taking us? *N Engl J Med.* Sep 19 1991;325(12):854–859.
6. Gilmer T, Kronick R, Rice T. Children welcome, adults need not apply: changes in public program enrollment across states and over time. *Med Care Res Rev.* Feb 2005; 62(1):56–78.
7. Kronick R, Gilmer T. Insuring low-income adults: does public coverage crowd out private? *Health Aff (Millwood).* Jan–Feb 2002;21(1):225–239.
8. Curtis R. Getting real about the uninsured problem. *Front Health Serv Manage.* Summer 2005;21(4):39–44; discussion 45–38.
9. Leape LL, Berwick DM. Five years after To Err Is Human: what have we learned? *JAMA.* May 18 2005;293(19):2384–2390.

10. Richardson WC, Berwick DM, Bisgard JC, et al. The Institute of Medicine Report on Medical Errors: misunderstanding can do harm. Quality of Health Care in America Committee. *MedGenMed.* Sep 19 2000;2(3):E42.
11. Woolf SH. United States Preventive Services Task Force recommendations on breast cancer screening. *Cancer.* Apr 1 1992;69(7 Suppl):1913–1918.
12. Berg AO, Allan J, Woolf S. The mammography dilemma. *Ann Intern Med.* May 6 2003;138(9):770–771; author reply 771.
13. Humphrey LL, Helfand M, Chan BK, Woolf SH. Breast cancer screening: a summary of the evidence for the U.S. Preventive Services Task Force. *Ann Intern Med.* Sep 3 2002;137(5 Part 1):347–360.
14. Eddy DM. Breast cancer screening in women younger than 50 years of age: what's next? *Ann Intern Med.* Dec 1 1997;127(11):1035–1036.
15. Reinhardt UE, Hussey PS, Anderson GF. U.S. health care spending in an international context. *Health Aff (Millwood).* May–Jun 2004;23(3):10–25.
16. Starfield B. Is US health really the best in the world? *J Am Med Assoc.* 2000;284(4):483–485.
17. Baicker K, Chandra A, Skinner JS. Geographic variation in health care and the problem of measuring racial disparities. *Perspect Biol Med.* Winter 2005;48(1 Suppl):S42–53.

Chapter 2
The Disease-Reservoir Hypothesis

Chapter 1 began with the story of Sally, a 77-year-old woman who had been diagnosed with ductal breast cancer. Sally received aggressive treatment and went on to live a life free of breast cancer. She also suffered from the consequences of the treatment. Not everyone believes that Sally required treatment, but few would advise her *against* taking action. The suggestion that Sally consider foregoing treatment disturbs many people. However, we do need to ask, what would happen if she consumed, and if we as a nation consumed, less medical care? The question is deceptively simple, but the answer maddeningly difficult.

To attempt an answer, it is best to begin at the beginning. The purpose of healthcare is to improve health. Health outcomes can be defined in terms of only two measurements: quantity of life and quality of life. A successful treatment is one that makes people live longer and/or improves quality of life [1, 2]. If a treatment neither extends life nor improves its quality, we must challenge whether it has benefit. Many people express their level of wellness in terms of numbers given by common medical tests, such as blood pressure, low-density lipoprotein (LDL) cholesterol, or blood sugar. These numbers have earned their importance because they are related to the chances of having a shorter life or of developing a disability or illness in the future. Other biological markers are less clearly related to meaningful clinical outcomes. Biomarkers such as measures of blood chemistry, cholesterol, or genetic typing should only be considered important if they are correlated with either quality or quantity of life.

It is becoming increasingly clear that there are also huge reservoirs of undiagnosed disease in human populations. As diagnostic technology improves, the healthcare system will be challenged because these common, previously undiagnosed problems will be identified in many individuals who may not benefit from treatment because their length of life or quality of life will never be affected. The problem has been fiercely debated in relation to cancer-screening tests such as mammography and prostate-specific antigen (PSA) [3, 4].

According to the American Cancer Society, screening and early detection of cancers save lives [5]. It is believed that there is an undetected reservoir of this disease that might be eliminated through more aggressive intervention.

R.M. Kaplan, *Disease, Diagnoses, and Dollars*, DOI 10.1007/978-0-387-74045-4_2,
© Springer Science+Business Media, LLC 2009

Screening guidelines have been proposed, and compliance to guidelines is now used as evidence for high-quality medical care [6]. Furthermore, test rates are increasing because there are now financial incentives for physicians to offer specific tests, such as mammography [7].

In order to better understand the problem, it is necessary to understand the natural history of disease. Public-health campaigns assume that disease is binary; either a person has the "diagnosis" or he does not. However, most diseases are processes. It is likely that chronic disease begins long before it is diagnosed. For example, autopsy studies consistently show that most young adults who died early in life from noncardiovascular causes have fatty streaks in their coronary arteries indicating the initiation of coronary disease [8]. Not all people who have a disease will ultimately suffer from the problem. With many diseases, most of those affected will never even know they are sick. For example, autopsy studies show that nearly half of men who die in their 70 s or 80 s have prostate cancer [9] and that nearly 40 percent of women in their 70 s had some evidence of breast cancer at the time they died [10]. However, most of these people were never tested for these cancers and never knew of these problems. Diagnosis and treatment could have resulted in complications but are unlikely to have improved health [3].

Among those who do have problems, some may not benefit from treatment. For example, if smokers are screened for lung cancer, many cases can be identified [11]. However, clinical trials have shown that the course of the disease is likely to be the same for those who are screened and those not subjected to screening, even though screening leads to more diagnosis and treatment [12]. The harder we look, the more likely it is that cases will be found. A very sensitive test for prostate cancer may detect disease in ten men; eventually one man will die of the disease. These problems are not limited to cancer. Advanced MRI technology has revealed surprisingly high rates of undiagnosed stroke. One cross-sectional study of 3,502 men and women over age 65 found that 29 percent had evidence of mild stokes and that 75 percent had plaque in their carotid arteries [13].

William Black and Gilbert Welch, who are professors at the Dartmouth Medical School, make the distinction between disease and pseudodisease [14]. Pseudodisease, in their description, is disease that will not affect life duration or quality of life. A diagnosis followed by surgical treatment may have consequences, often leaving the patient with new -symptoms or problems. The study of what happens to patients in terms of life expectancy and patient experiences is called outcomes research.

Outcomes researchers consider the benefits of screening and treatment from the patient's perspective [15]. Using information provided by patients, quality of life and mortality outcomes are combined into quality-adjusted life years (QALYs). QALYs are estimated to evaluate whether patients are better off with or without screening and treatment [16]. The concept of QALYs will be described in great detail in Chapter 9.

What Is Disease?

The Merriam-Webster dictionary defines disease as "a condition of the living animal or plant body or of one of its parts that impairs normal functioning and is typically manifested by distinguishing signs and symptoms." Disease, quite literally, is the lack of ease. It is apparent when there is dysfunction or symptoms.

The dictionary definition of disease raises several important questions. Do we have disease if there is not dysfunction, symptoms, or a lack of ease? In other words, what do we do about conditions that do not cause signs or symptoms? The answer is fairly clear. Pathological conditions that will cause signs or symptoms at some future time must qualify as disease. For example, high blood pressure is associated with the increased probability of stroke or heart attacks in the future [17]. Even though a condition does not cause symptoms or dysfunction now, it must be of concern if somewhere down the road it will cause early death, dysfunction, or other symptoms. And let us take this one step further. Suppose that a condition does not cause symptoms or dysfunction now and it will never cause early death, dysfunction, or symptoms. Does the condition then qualify as a disease?

In modern medicine, we know of many conditions that represent genuine pathology of a tissue but may never cause early death, dysfunction, or symptoms. In fact, this may be so for the majority of cases of prostate cancer [18]. In addition, the substantial majority of cases of low-grade breast cancer (ductal carcinoma in situ) would never affect people's lives if they had not been diagnosed. Autopsy studies suggest as many as 60 percent of men die with prostate cancer while only about 3 percent of men die of prostate cancer. Similarly, autopsy studies have shown that nearly 40 percent of older women may have ductile carcinoma in situ (DCIS) at the time of death. However, only about 3 percent of women die of breast cancer [10].

These observations suggest that the reservoir of undiagnosed disease is quite large. Doing more tests significantly increases the number of cases that will be detected. Not only are we doing more tests; inevitably, as medicine and technology march on, new tests become available, and more often than not the new tests are much more sensitive and accurate than the old ones. But the question is, are they *better*—that is, do they actually result in better outcomes for patients? There is a lot of debate about how many doctors and how many tests are necessary. Between 1975 and 1995, the number of cardiologists doubled and the number of radiologists increased five-fold [19]. After the mid-1990 s, training programs began to reduce the number of cardiologists and radiologists in training. For cardiology, the peak year was 1995, when there were 2,354 fellows in training programs. By 2003, the number had been reduced to 2,117 [20]. Similarly, the number of radiologists in training slowed in the last decade. However, both the cardiology and the radiology professions argue that there will be a serious shortage of diagnostic specialists in the future

[21, 22]. At least two factors account for this problem. First, the demographics of the population suggest that a higher proportion of all people will be elderly and in need of these diagnostic services. Second, diagnostic sub-specialties have new tools that make them more valuable. So, it is likely that we will soon see another increase in "diagnosis-heavy" or testing-heavy specialists. In fact, this problem has been made worse by payment schedules. While primary care doctors struggle to make ends meet, physicians specializing in testing and diagnosis have seen their relative incomes rise.

With more doctors having expertise in diagnosis and with better diagnostic technologies, we are discovering that more people are sick. For example, new spiral CT scans can detect hepatic lesions (lesions of the liver) that are less than 2 mm. In 1982, the smallest lesions that could be detected were 20 mm. Studies now suggest that MRI can detect abnormalities in the knees of 25 percent of healthy young men. When MRI is applied to the back, bulging discs are detected in 50 percent of adults, even though most of these adults do not have back pain. By age 50–59, 4 in 5 adults will have a bulging disc, even though there is no corresponding increase in the incidence of back pain. Figure 2.1 shows that the proportion of people with bulging discs increases systematically with age [23]. The two lines on the figure represent two different observers. Different radiologists do not see the pictures exactly the same, and the figure reflects this difference in judgment. However, the judgment of the two doctors is very similar.

Even though the rate of diagnosis is very high, it is expected to go even high as medical technology improves. The most recent advance is electron beam computerized tomography or CT. Using these methods, a healthy person can have their whole body scanned. This "whole body scanning" has become popular in nontraditional settings. Radio and television advertisements encourage people to go to a nonhospital free standing center to be scanned for problems they might even suspect. When applied to groups with moderate risk, a remarkably high percentage is identified as having a problem. For

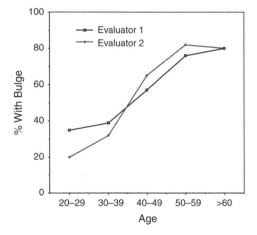

Fig. 2.1 Percent of disk bulges discovered by Magnetic Resonance Imaging (MRI) in volunteers without back pain (Jensen et al. [23])

example, 75 percent of adults who undergo full body screening end up with additional diagnostic work up and about half of patients who get scanning for calcium in the coronary arteries end up with additional tests.

Surveys show that most adults in the USA rate their health status as excellent or good. However, diagnostic tests, especially many advanced and "whole-body" tests, suggest that very few of us are truly well. In fact, virtually all of us have some kind of a problem that can be detected with modern medical technology. But what does this mean in terms of how individuals should behave in seeking out medical treatment? And what does it mean in terms of how we as a society should invest in healthcare? What I propose is that we consider a new way to think about these personal and social questions about healthcare, and I summarize this new way of thinking in a single sentence: *It may be okay to be sick.*

Coming from a management professional in healthcare, that statement may sound hard-hearted or even crazy, but it is neither. In many cases, we are sick with pseudodisease rather than with true disease. In other words, problems that were once hidden but that we are now able to detect often turn out to be those that never cause symptoms, disability, or early death. One of the challenges we face and will increasingly face is that newer and better diagnostic techniques are only going to make this problem worse. It might be argued that advances in diagnostic technology actually produce harm because they identify pseudodisease rather than real disease. Among people diagnosed with pseudodisease, many will get additional tests and treatment. Some of these treatments result in complications that ultimately reduce quality of life. Older men with prostate cancer, for example, are most likely to complete their lives with no complications from their illness. Newer technologies that diagnose the problem may lead to treatments, which in turn may cause impotence or incontinence. Treatments sometimes do good, and even save lives, but we also must be aware that treatments can produce harm. The challenge is to know when to pursue treatment and when to leave well enough alone. To even begin to discuss the options, we have to take a look at the numbers.

Testing the Disease-Reservoir Hypothesis

According to the disease-reservoir process, the more we look for disease, the more likely we are to find it. Table 2.1, based on a *New England Journal of Medicine* article by Black and Welch [25] summarizes the percentages of people in the USA who die from breast cancer, prostate cancer, or thyroid cancer. The

Table 2.1 What percentage of people have cancer?

Site	Deaths (%)	Autopsy (%)
Breast	3.0	39
Prostate	3.0	46
Thyroid	0.1	100

table also summarizes the rate at which these cancers are discovered at autopsy in at least some studies. About 3 percent of women die of breast cancer and 3 percent of men die of prostate cancer. Thyroid cancer is a relatively rare cause of death. It accounts for about 0.1 percent of all fatalities. However, autopsy studies show that large numbers of people who died of other causes have cancer that was never known to them. For example, for older women who die of noncancer causes some studies have shown that as many as 39 percent have some form of breast cancer [3] and nearly half of men who die of noncancer deaths actually had prostate cancer and never knew it. The most striking finding is for atypical cells in the thyroid. This condition will effect us all by our mid-70 s. However, these atypical cancer-like cells in our thyroid glands will effect only one person in a thousand (Black & Welch).

The disease-reservoir hypothesis argues that the more we look for disease, the more likely we are to find it. If disease is there to be found, being aggressive in the search will turn up evidence. And sure enough, Welch and colleagues reported evidence using the number of slides per woman taken at autopsy and the probability of identification of ductal breast cancer. There is a systematic relationship positive correlation between the number of slides taken for examination and the likelihood that the woman is diagnosed with breast cancer (see Table 2.2). With only nine slides per woman, the DCIS rate has been reported to be close to 0 percent. However, in studies using 275 sample slides per woman, the rate of DCIS has been as high as 39 percent [10].

The connection between diagnosis and treatment raises several important issues. Since diagnoses typically lead to further treatment, people living in areas with high rates of diagnostic testing are more likely to get further workups for health conditions. Kaplan and Saltzstein [26] considered the problem of declining cancer rates among the oldest members of society. The study considered two issues. First, it asked how many women in each age group were diagnosed with cancer in situ (CIS). These are cases of cancer that are well confined and have not spread. The rate of diagnoses of breast cancer increases with age until about age 75. Thereafter, identification of new breast cancer systematically declines with age. This raises some interesting questions. Could it be that once women reach their mid-70 s, their bodies resist cancer? Probably not. As noted above, autopsy studies show high rates of undiagnosed cancers in the bodies of women who died after age 75. Another explanation for the decline in cancer cases is that doctors stop looking for cancer in older women. The Kaplan and Saltzstein

Table 2.2 Prevalence of Ductile Carcinoma in situ (DCIS) by number of slides per women in four different studies

Reference	Slides	% DCIS
Bartow et al., 1987	9	0
Kramer et al., 1973	40	4.3
Neilsen et al., 1984	95	14.3
Neilson et al., 1987	275	39

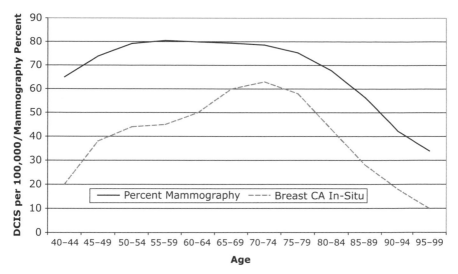

Fig. 2.2 Mammography and breast carcinoma in situ (CIS) by age. (Adapted from data in Kaplan and Saltzstein [26])

study also showed that the use of mammography increases until about age 75 and systematically declines in a manner parallel to the rate of known new breast cancer cases (see Fig. 2.2) [27].

The Geographic Distribution of Health Services

Another implication of the disease-reservoir hypothesis is that demand for health services is elastic. Since disease is common, it will be found when physicians look for it, and more will be found when they look harder. Yet, much of what is found is pseudodisease. Finding more will not necessarily result in better health outcomes. This conflicts with our traditional belief that most treatment is necessary.

We have always assumed that if a doctor diagnoses a disease, that disease exists. Furthermore, we assume that any two (or three or six) qualified doctors presented with the same problem will come to the same diagnosis. Keen observers are aware that there will be variability. Professionals make errors in diagnosis, but we assume that these errors are random. Thus, if the true distribution of disease is the same in different communities, we would expect the rates of reporting to be roughly equivalent. However, physicians are very different in the rates of illness they detect and in the services they recommend. Wennberg and his colleagues have devoted the past quarter century to the description of this problem [28, 29]. Wennberg suggests that a major factor in the use of medical services is "supplier-induced demand." This implies that providers create demand for their services by diagnosing illnesses. When new diagnostic technologies gain acceptance from physician groups, new epidemics of "disease" appear. One of the earliest documented cases of supplier-induced demand was described by Glover in the UK. Glover (cited by Wennberg [30]) recorded the rates of tonsillectomy in the Hornse Burrough school district. In 1928, 186 children in the district had their tonsils surgically removed. The next year, the doctor who enthusiastically supported tonsillectomy was replaced by another physician who was less attracted to the procedure. In 1929, the number of tonsillectomies declined to only 12.

Supplier-induced demand does not apply the procedures that are really necessary. In most surgical subspecialties, surgeons would agree on the need to perform surgery for some well-defined cases. These might include amputation of a toe with gangrene, removal of some well-defined tumors, or intervention to repair a compound fracture. However, for most surgical procedures, there is substantial discretion in the determination of need for surgery. In these cases, the number of surgeries may be related to the number of surgeons.

A Case Study

Boston, Massachusetts, and New Haven, Connecticut, are similar in a variety of ways. Both are traditional New England cities with multiethnic populations. The two cities have approximately the same climate, and both cities are home to prestigious Ivy-League universities, including distinguished medical schools. Since the cities are near one another, we would expect their costs for medical care to be approximately the same. Using data from the mid-1970 s, Wennberg and colleagues [30] demonstrated that, in fact, medical care in Boston costs nearly twice as much as in New Haven.

In 1975, Medicare paid $324.00 per recipient per month for people in Boston and only $155.00 per month for residents of New Haven. The situation has not changed much. In 1989, per-capita hospital expenditures for acute care were $1,524 for residents of Boston and $777 for those living in New Haven. By 2000, medical care in the USA had changed, but most differences between practice in Boston and New Haven remained. One of the reasons that Boston and New Haven differ in cost is that patients are significantly more likely to be readmitted to the hospital for the same conditions in Boston. Figure 2.3 shows the comparison of readmissions between Boston and New Haven in 2000. Patients in Boston are readmitted 1.64 times for each time equivalent patients are readmitted in New Haven. For cancer surgery readmissions, Boston patients are readmitted 81 percent more often than New Haven patients.

Further study by Wennberg and his colleagues showed that Boston has more hospital capacity than does New Haven [31]. In Boston, there are 4.3 hospital beds for every 1,000 residents, while in New Haven there are fewer than 2.3 beds per 1,000 residents. Residents of Boston are more likely to be hospitalized for a wide variety of acute medical conditions than are residents of New Haven. For a variety of medical conditions, such as pneumonia or congestive heart failure,

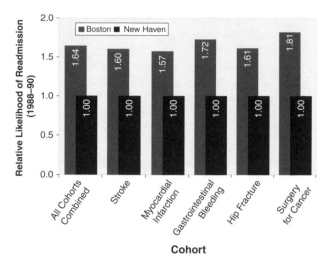

Fig. 2.3 Difference in Medicare expenditures between Boston and New Haven

Bostonians are more likely to be cared for as hospital inpatients, while residents of New Haven tend to be treated outside the hospital [28].

Boston is rich with medical institutions. New Haven has only one major medical school (Yale), while Boston has three (Harvard, Boston University, and Tufts). Furthermore, the Harvard Medical School is associated with a variety of different teaching hospitals. Boston has four hospitals associated with different religious establishments, while there is only one religiously affiliated hospital in New Haven.

The Boston vs. New Haven comparison is particularly interesting from a public-policy perspective. The US Medicare is a federal program meant to provide equal benefit to all of its recipients. In the 1970 s, Medicare was spending twice as much in Boston as it did in New Haven [30]. The question must be asked, were New Haven residents getting a bad deal? Since the government was spending less on New Haven residents, it might be argued that their health should suffer. However, evidence does not show that residents of Boston are any healthier than residents of New Haven. In fact, some evidence implies that Boston residents may be worse off. As noted above people in Boston are more likely to be re-hospitalized for the same condition than people in New Haven [32]. Residents of Boston appear to have more complications from medical treatment. More may not necessarily be better. Indeed, there is some suggestive evidence that more may be worse [33, 32].

Studies of Regional Variation in Service and Spending

In 2005, an estimated $2 trillion was spent for hospital care in the USA. In other words, we spent more than $6,700 per person on health care (the data is from the US Center for Health Statistics) [34]. Of course, that amount was not spent on each individual. You may not have been hospitalized in 2005, but some people were hospitalized for extended periods or for services that were very expensive. Averages do not tell us much about individual cases.

Still, there are important lessons to be learned by looking at the overall expenditures data for different locales. Within the USA, we would expect the average costs to be similar in regions serving an equal number of people. Yet that is not the case. For most of my career I worked at the medical school at the University of California, San Diego. A few years ago, I moved to the University of California, Los Angeles. My physical move took me only about 100 miles, and the communities are demographically very similar. However, the differences in how medicine is practiced are surprisingly different. Using the most recent data in 2006, Medicare was spending an average of $11,639 per recipient in Los Angeles and $6,654 in San Diego for services offered during the last two years of life. In other words, Medicare is spending $1.75 in Los Angeles to purchase the same package of services that they spend $1.00 just 120 miles down the road. A summary of variation in spending is shown in Fig. 2.4. Differences between total Medicare (Parts A and B) 2005 expenditures in San Diego and Los Angeles health services areas are summarized in Fig. 2.4. The lowest cost Los Angeles health service area (Torrence) was more expensive than the highest cost community (La Mesa) in San Diego County. Considering Los Angeles as a benchmark, Glendale, had 2005 expenditures that were 97% of those in Los Angeles. The most expensive San Diego community of La Mesa, had mean per recipient expenditures that were 69% of what was spent per recipient in Los Angeles. The San Diego County community of La Jolla, had expenditures that were only half of those in Los Angeles. There was very little overlap between

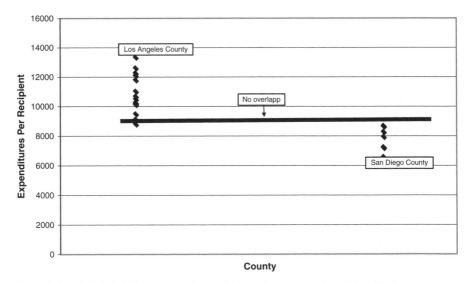

Fig. 2.4 Total 2005 Medicare expenditures in Los Angeles and San Diego HSAs

the San Diego and the Los Angeles markets for total Medical reimbursements, total Part A expenditures, total Part B expenditures, percent of Medicare deaths occurring within a hospital, inpatient hospital reimbursement, hospital admission during the last six months of life, Part B reimbursements to physicians, and reimbursements for professional and laboratory services.

The analysis of Medicare claims has an important methodological advantage over virtually any other database because Medicare pays for healthcare for essentially all individuals 65 years or older. The analyses use essentially the entire claims data base or a representative 5 percent sample. These include hundreds of millions of claims, so the usual sources of sampling error are essentially absent from these analyses. What is most striking about these studies is that the amount of healthcare delivered in different geographic regions is highly variable. Some regions get much more than others. However, we have very little evidence that those living in areas that receive more care have better health outcomes than those living in areas that receive less care.

Variation and Cost

Many medical conditions are associated with higher prevalence and treatment than others, as shown on the map. For example, there is not large variation in treatment options for problems such as fracture of the hip. Patients who fracture their hips are likely to be admitted to the hospital wherever they live. However, the Dartmouth group estimates that 80 percent of patients who are admitted to hospitals have been diagnosed with high-variation medical conditions, such as pneumonia, chronic obstructive pulmonary disease, gastroenteritis, and congestive heart failure. They argue that hospital capacity has a major influence on the likelihood that a patient will be hospitalized. This relationship is illustrated in Fig. 2.5. The figure shows the relationship between hospital beds per 1,000 residents and hospitalization for high-variation medical conditions. The correlation between hospital beds and admissions is a remarkable 0.76. In hospital-referral regions where there are fewer than 2.5 beds per 1,000 residents, the hospital discharge rate for high-variation conditions was 145 per 1,000. Among regions that had more than 4.5 beds per 1,000 residents, the rate was 219.8. In other words, more beds means more hospitalizations. These data argue that the decision to admit a patient to the hospital is influenced by factors other than the patient's medical condition. When beds are available, they are more likely to be used. When more hospital beds are used, healthcare costs go up.

The number of beds best predicts medical care use for medical admissions. As Fig. 2.5 suggests, the relationship is weaker for surgical admissions. The bottom line on the figure shows the relationship for hip fracture. This is an interesting case because there is little discretion in the decision to hospitalize someone for hip fracture. When hospitalization is truly necessary, as in the case

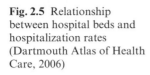

Fig. 2.5 Relationship between hospital beds and hospitalization rates (Dartmouth Atlas of Health Care, 2006)

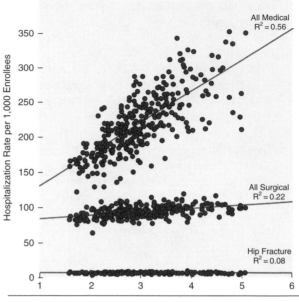

Hospital Beds per 1,000 residents of HRRs

of that condition, the number of beds available no longer predicts the number of hospitalization rates.

It seems plausible that communities with greater hospital resources are better able to care for their populations. More healthcare should lead to more health. However, several analyses have shown that people are slightly more likely to die in communities where more acute hospital care is used [33]. The obvious explanation is that these communities have people who are older, sicker, or poorer. Careful analyses controlling for age, sex, race, income, and a variety of variables related to illness and the need for care have been carried out. None of these variables was able to explain the relationship. In other words, the analysis suggests that more is not better. In fact, it implies that more may be worse [33, 35].

References

1. Kaplan RM, Wingard DL. Trends in breast cancer incidence, survival, and mortality. *Lancet.* Aug 12 2000;356(9229):592–593.
2. Kaplan RM. The Ziggy Theorem – toward an Outcomes-Focused Health Psychology. *Health Psychol.* 1994;13(6):451–460.
3. Welch HG, Black WC. Using autopsy series to estimate the disease "reservoir" for ductal carcinoma in situ of the breast: how much more breast cancer can we find? *Ann Intern Med.* Dec 1 1997;127(11):1023–1028.
4. Welch HG, Schwartz LM, Woloshin S. Do increased 5-year survival rates in prostate cancer indicate better outcomes? *JAMA.*Oct 25 2000;284(16):2053–2055.

5. Kaplan RM, Groessl EJ. Cost/effectiveness analysis in behavioral medicine. *J Consult Clin Psychol*.2002; in press.
6. McGlynn EA, Asch SM, Adams J, et al. The quality of health care delivered to adults in the United States. *N Engl J Med*.Jun 26 2003;348(26):2635–2645.
7. Epstein AM, Lee TH, Hamel MB. Paying physicians for high-quality care. *N Engl J Med*. Jan 22 2004;350(4):406–410.
8. Strong JP, Malcom GT, McMahan CA, et al. Prevalence and extent of atherosclerosis in adolescents and young adults: implications for prevention from the Pathobiological Determinants of Atherosclerosis in Youth Study. *JAMA*.1999;281(8):727–735.
9. Gosselaar C, Roobol MJ, Schroder FH. Prevalence and characteristics of screen-detected prostate carcinomas at low prostate-specific antigen levels: aggressive or insignificant? *BJU Int*.Feb 2005;95(2):231–237.
10. Welch HG, Black WC. Using autopsy series to estimate the disease "reservoir" for ductal carcinoma in situ of the breast: how much more breast cancer can we find? *Ann Intern Med*.1997;127(11):1023–1028.
11. Klingler K. Early dection of lung cancer by CT-screening. *Eur J Cancer: ECJ Suppl.* 2004;2(1):23.
12. Marcus PM, Bergstralh EJ, Fagerstrom RM, et al. Lung cancer mortality in the Mayo Lung Project: impact of extended follow-up. *J Natl Cancer Inst*.Aug 16 2000; 92(16):1308–1316.
13. Manolio TA, Burke GL, O'Leary DH, et al. Relationships of cerebral MRI findings to ultrasonographic carotid atherosclerosis in older adults: the Cardiovascular Health Study. CHS Collaborative Research Group. *Arterioscler Thromb Vasc Biol.* 1999;19(2):356–365.
14. Black WC, Welch HG. Screening for disease. *AJR. Am J Roentgenol*.1997;168(1):3–11.
15. Kaplan RM. Two pathways to prevention. *Am Psychol*.Apr 2000;55(4):382–396.
16. Kaplan RM. Decisions about prostate cancer screening in managed care. *Curr Opin Oncol*.1997;9(5):480–486.
17. MacMahon S. Blood pressure and the risk of cardiovascular disease. *N Engl J Med*.Jan 6 2000;342(1):50–52.
18. Black WC. Should this patient be screened for cancer? *Eff Clin Pract*.Mar–Apr 1999;2(2):86–95.
19. Fisher ES, Welch HG. Avoiding the unintended consequences of growth in medical care: how might more be worse? *JAMA*.1999;281(5):446–453.
20. Fye WB. Cardiology workforce: a shortage, not a surplus. *Health Aff (Millwood)*. Jan–Jun 2004;Suppl Web Exclusives:W4-64–W4-66.
21. Bhargavan M, Sunshine JH, Schepps B. Data from a professional society placement service as a measure of the employment market for radiation oncologists. *Int J Radiat Oncol Biol Phys*.Jun 1 2002;53(2):401–406.
22. Bhargavan M, Sunshine JH, Schepps B. Too few radiologists? *AJR Am J Roentgenol*.May 2002;178(5):1075–1082.
23. Jensen MC, Brant-Zawadzki MN, Obuchowski N, Modic MT, Malkasian D, Ross JS. Magnetic resonance imaging of the lumbar spine in people without back pain. *N Engl J Med*.Jul 14 1994;331(2):69–73.
24. Hunold P, Schmermund A, Seibel RM, Gronemeyer DH, Erbel R. Prevalence and clinical significance of accidental findings in electron-beam tomographic scans for coronary artery calcification. *Eur Heart* J. 2001;22:1748–1758.
25. Black WC, Welch HG. Advances in diagnostic imaging and overestimations of disease prevalence and the benefits of therapy. *N Engl J Med*. 1993;328(17):1237–1243.
26. Kaplan RM, Saltzstein SL. Reduced mammographic screening may explain declines in breast carcinoma in older women. *J Am Geriatr Soc*.May 2005;53(5):862–866.
27. Kaplan RM, Ganiats TG, Frosch DL. Diagnostic and treatment decisions in US health-care. *J Health Psychol*.Jan 2004;9(1):29–40.

28. Wennberg JE. *The Dartmouth Atlas of Health Care in the United States.* Hanover, NH: Trustees of Dartmouth College; 1998.
29. Wennberg JE, Fisher ES, Skinner JS. Geography and the debate over Medicare reform. *Health Aff (Millwood)*.2002;Suppl Web Exclusives:W96–114.
30. Wennberg JE. Small area analysis and the medical care outcome problem. Paper presented at: Research Methodology: Strengthening Causal Interpretations of Nonexperimental Data, 1990; Rockville, MD.
31. Wennberg J, Gittelsohn A. Variations in medical care among small areas. *Sci Am.* 1982;246(4):120–134.
32. Fisher ES, Wennberg JE, Stukel TA, Sharp S. Hospital readmissions rates for cohorts of Medicare beneficiaries in Boston and New Haven. *N Engl J Med.*1994;331(15):989–995.
33. Fisher ES, Wennberg DE, Stukel TA, Gottlieb DJ, Lucas FL, Pinder EL. The implications of regional variations in Medicare spending. Part 1: the content, quality, and accessibility of care. *Ann Intern Med.*Feb 18 2003;138(4):273–287.
34. Smith C, Cowan C, Sensenig A, Catlin A. Health spending growth slows in 2003. *Health Aff (Millwood)*.Jan–Feb 2005;24(1):185–194.
35. Fisher ES, Welch HG. Could more health care lead to worse health? *Hosp Pract (Off Ed)*. Nov 15 1999;34(12):15–16, 21–12, 25 passim.

Chapter 3
Mental Models of Health and Healthcare

Modern biology, physiology, and anatomy have done wonders for our understanding of disease. New techniques in radiology allow visualization of even minor anatomical defects. Contemporary laboratory methods offer advanced diagnoses of countless major and minor illnesses. The scientific basis for understanding disease has never been better. In the last decade, our insights into the basic mechanisms of disease have advanced at an incredible pace, and there is every reason to believe that the breadth and depth of our understanding will continue to grow at an extremely rapid rate.

Beliefs about the basis of disease guide decisions about medical intervention. But they also influence personal health decisions and public-health policies, investment and research agendas in private corporations and academic institutions, and government funding as well as donations to charities for a wide variety of healthcare delivery and medical research programs. Our beliefs about or mental representations of disease are sometimes called "illness models," or just "models." Before our modern understanding of disease, models that we now joke about dominated medical thinking. The Greek philosopher Hippocrates (460–377 BC) described four basic temperaments, known as "humors," in relation to physical characteristics. These ideas were expanded by the Greek-born Roman physician Claudius Galen (129–216 BC), who believed that all diseases were caused by imbalances between the four humors, and that the humors were related to personality characteristics as well as bodily fluids. The *sanguine* humor, derived from blood, was connected with a cheerful, confident, and optimistic temperament. *Choleric* humor, believed to be physiologically derived from yellow bile, was associated with an easily angered temperament. *Black bile* was believed to be the root of a depressed temperament and melancholic personality. Calm, sluggish, and unemotional temperaments were believed to result from *phlegm,* or the phlegmatic humor. Galen constantly did detailed studies in anatomy and physiology, reportedly employing 20 scribes to help document his findings, and his influence was enormous and long-lasting. For nearly 1,500 years, his teachings formed the basis of medicine and medical care in most of the Western world. It was not until the seventeenth century that Vesalius, an anatomist from northern Europe who also lived in France and Italy, began to disassemble Galen's dictums. Galen's scientific

R.M. Kaplan, *Disease, Diagnoses, and Dollars*, DOI 10.1007/978-0-387-74045-4_3,
© Springer Science+Business Media, LLC 2009

observations were detailed, systematic, and credible, but they were also wrong in many important ways. They fed mental models of illness that misled western physicians and other healers for centuries—including most of our recorded history.

Among all the wrongheaded notions about disease in premodern medicine, perhaps the most dramatic were those relating to mental problems. For centuries, it was believed that what we call mental illness resulted from possession by demons. Brutal approaches were used to rid sufferers from the spirits that controlled their behaviors and emotions. But as easy as it is to be flabbergasted or appalled by primitive reactions to "possession," even today many health decisions are influenced by, and sometimes thwarted by, traditional cultural beliefs. A fascinating book by Anne Fadiman documents the struggle of a Laotian family, members of the Hmong tribe, caught between their traditional beliefs about their child's chronic illness and an American healthcare system ill-equipped to grapple with the problem. *The Spirit Catches You and You Fall Down* chronicles the story of a child with epilepsy. At 3 months of age she had a seizure, which her family believed had resulted from the slamming of their home's front door by an older sister. In their culture, seizures were regarded as a sign of wisdom. They believed that the young child's soul had left her body and become lost to a different guiding spirit. Highly trained American doctors in California, the family's adopted home, of course worked on the young girl's case based on a modern medical mental model of illness, with a set of assumptions and treatments completely different from that of the family's. In the end, because of repeated mishandling and miscommunication, largely the result of a thorough-going cultural disconnect, the child was seriously harmed by overmedication and died by the age of 7. Of course, mental models of disease can also enhance understanding, insight, and practice. They are by no means always, or even mostly, an impediment to sound diagnoses and beneficial treatment. The point here, though, is their power. Models direct decisions about how we care for ourselves and for others. What may seem logical and credible to one culture might be unacceptable to another. Knowledge about the mechanisms of disease continually evolves, and it is likely that many of our current conceptualizations will require modification.

New data may even force us to abruptly revise one of our mental models of illness. A personal example may help illustrate the point. For various reasons, I believed that extracts of Echinacea roots could be used to treat or prevent the common cold. Echinacea was a common remedy among Native Americans and has been used as a treatment for the common cold for more than 100 years. The mechanism was believed to work through the up-regulation of the immune system and inflammatory responses. For several years, I swallowed Echinacea pills each time I experienced the early symptoms of a cold. I was not alone. Echinacea was used by literally millions of people around the world. However, Turner and colleagues [1] eventually conducted a randomized clinical trial to systematically evaluate the benefits of Echinacea. The results suggested that Echinacea has absolutely no effects on established infections or on the prevention of the common cold. I wanted to disbelieve the results, but the study was so well designed and executed that I have been forced to alter my mental model. The following winter I went without Echinacea and also went cold-free.

The Human Body: Component Parts or Systems?

The art of medicine concentrates on diagnosis (finding problems) and treatment (fixing problems). Put at its simplest, the task of physicians might be described as "find it and fix it." The find-it-fix-it model exemplifies what engineers call linear thinking. The linear model has been the predominant view of the universe since the time of Sir Isaac Newton, who focused his attention on discrete components of the universe and analyzed how these components existed independently of one another but had cause-and-effect relationships. Many things work in a linear fashion. The environment receives relatively little attention. Ackoff [2] explained that the industrial revolution, which began in England in the eighteenth century, ushered in new ways of thinking that dominated nearly all fields for several centuries. This thinking was built on the foundation of three linear-model concepts: reductionism, analysis, and mechanism.

Reductionism is a belief that anything we experience or investigate can be better understood by examining its component parts. Just as an automobile is made up of thousands of individual parts, we assume that human beings are also a conglomeration of parts, and that by examining these parts individually, we can better understand how the body functions or malfunctions.

Analysis is the process by which things are divided into their components. These things may be tangible, such as the human body or a machine. However, ideas can also be disassembled.

Mechanism, the third basic component of linear thinking, is the belief that cause and effect can be described by one relationship. If x causes y, we may understand the mechanism of y by manipulating x.

Understanding complexity is a fundamental goal of science. In the nineteenth century, Descartes proposed reductionism as a remedy to being overwhelmed by information. According to Descartes, complicated phenomena could be understood by dividing them into their component parts. It was assumed that this division would not distort the phenomenon that was being studied. This approach has led to many productive advances in science. It is also apparent, however, that there are dense interconnections among the component parts of most phenomena and that linear models do not always tell the whole story. Virtually all sciences have come to this same conclusion [3].

A recent and increasingly popular alternative to linear thinking is "systems" thinking, which emphasizes consideration of the whole rather than the individual parts. A system is defined as a whole; it is not divided into independent parts. The functioning of each part cannot profitably be understood independent of the functioning of other parts. Understanding the value of individual parts is lost when the whole is disassembled [4].

Traditional scientific analysis represents an attempt to understand organisms by taking them apart and examining each part separately. This type of linear-model analysis is often very useful in determining the *structure* of an organism, but it very often will not supply us with much information about *function*. The traditional find-it-fix-it medical model builds upon traditional linear thinking. If a prostate gland is too large, it must be surgically reduced, high blood pressure must be lowered, and hyperactive children must be made less active. Certainly, mechanistic thinking has produced some sensational successes. Many patients benefit from hernia repairs, total joint replacement, and the pharmaceutical control of blood pressure. However, finding and fixing one problem often creates a new problem. Easy solutions, even those derived from understanding of basic mechanisms of disease, might set off or open the door to new problems. The human body is made up of highly complex systems, and intrusion into any one system is likely to affect other systems. Lung disease, for example, may affect the kidneys, the heart, and the circulatory systems. The systems are all connected and cannot be understood independently of one another.

The difference between linear and system thinking goes beyond basic physiology. It also applies to entire systems of healthcare. For example, because a healthcare system is a complex set of interconnections, tinkering with one component may have consequences for other components of the system. In later chapters, we will see that public policies designed to attend to one problem might create problems elsewhere. For example, well-intended policies designed to expand health insurance coverage for preventive health services may result in increased premiums for health insurance, which in turn may result in the loss of healthcare insurance for many people because some employers might choose, in light of the increased expense, to discontinue offering insurance for their employees. So the initial impulse to increase the number of people covered might end up actually reducing the number covered.

Chronic versus Acute Disease

Linear models of human diseases can in some cases be very misleading and result in inappropriate treatment decisions For example, it was once believed that people who had high levels of protein in their urine were in need of more protein in their diet—the logic being that they had to replace the protein lost in the process of excretion. Today, we know that exactly the opposite course of treatment is what is really needed: People with kidney disease, which often results in high levels of protein in their urine—need to avoid high levels of dietary protein. Similarly, people with back problems were once told to avoid any activity. The result was atrophy in other muscle groups and an increased chance of dangerous blood clots. Today, there a few conditions for which total bed rest is advised. The shortcomings of linear models can even apply to illness in general: The predominant belief that most diseases have a remedy should in all likelihood be scaled back, because in many cases leaving well enough alone is as effective as the best medicines.

The twentieth century saw remarkable advances in medicine and medical care, but many challenges remain at the beginning of the third millennium. The enemies of the modern physician have changed. One of the major accomplishments of traditional linear-model medicine has been the reduction of deaths from infectious diseases, at least in the industrialized world. Today, people in developed societies rarely die of tuberculosis, smallpox, and polio, which not too many decades ago were killers feared by everyone. Instead, now most of the challenges in the industrialized world come from chronic illnesses. These diseases require people to adapt and modify their lifestyles, meaning that much of our healthcare effort has had to switch from a curing model to a caring model. This may require new thinking about the definitions of health and healthcare.

Contemporary healthcare developed in the course of the twentieth century to attend to acute diseases, which typically were diagnosed and then treated (though sometimes patients would get better on their own). Confirming the diagnosis of an acute illness often involves a biological test done in a laboratory; patient reports about symptoms are often downplayed or disregarded as unreliable. Over the last five decades in economically advanced societies, the acute disease model has pretty much determined the planning and constructions of hospitals and laboratories, the development of training programs, and the creation of medical subspecialties [5]. However, the acute disease model now has significant limitations because the major patient population burden on our healthcare system has shifted from acute to chronic disease, but our systems for care have not kept up.

Chronic diseases typically have multiple causes, and people who have one chronic condition typically have other chronic diseases as well. The Medical Outcomes Study was a major effect to understand the long-term health consequences of common chronic diseases. The study began by recruiting patients who had one of six chronic diseases. For example, there was a hypertension sample, a chronic lung disease sample, and so on. However, over 90 percent of the participants in the study had at least one additional chronic condition—above and beyond the one they represented in the study [6].

Chronic diseases present other challenges. In contrast to acute diseases, which typically last for a relatively brief interval of time, chronic conditions are, by definition, usually not cured. As a result, patients must adapt to the problems brought on by the disease for prolonged periods of time, and psychological and social factors are often of key importance. Patients' interpretation of the condition and adaptation to the problem cannot be ignored.

A different conceptual model, referred to as the outcomes model [7], is needed to measure the consequences of chronic illness. In contrast to the traditional biomedical model, which requires identification of a basic disease mechanism, the outcomes model emphasizes all behavioral and social as well as physical consequences of the patient's condition. Sometimes, the exact biological determinants are unknown. While some people believe no medical treatments are of value unless the biological pathway underlying the disease is understood, the outcomes model recognizes that biologic pathways may never, in the case of some chronic conditions, be fully understood [8]. Furthermore, some behavioral risk factors affect health outcomes through a variety of different biological pathways. For example, researchers spent years attempting to identify the impact of tobacco use upon specific organs. Separate studies presented the effects of cigarette smoking on lung cancer, heart disease, emphysema, oral cancers, and so on. By looking at the disease-specific impact of smoking and emphasizing the specific biological models, the total impact of tobacco use was underestimated. The outcomes approach links tobacco use to deaths from all causes and to reductions in quality of life. Considered from this perspective, the impact of tobacco use is huge, accounting for an estimated 19 percent of all premature death [9]. Taken in its totality with the outcomes model, tobacco use is far and away the leading cause of preventable death in the USA.

Common-Sense Models

Many decisions about healthcare are based on common-sense models, which describe the ways patients conceptualize their own illness. The models are based on understandings of the illness that result from *experience* of the symptoms, as well as other life experiences. These common-sense models often differ significantly from the biomedical views of illness.

Studies indicate that the way patients conceptualize their illness is important in determining the distress that they experience. For example, one study evaluated 69 breast cancer patients before and after treatment. The assessment that was conducted before treatment included extensive information about stress and the way that the patients conceptualized their cancer. Those who thought of their cancer as chronic or relapsing reported more anxiety, depression, and worry about recurrence than those who thought of their cancer as an acute illness. These belief patterns affected the way that the patients went about their treatment. Not surprisingly, mental models are important in guiding patients' treatment choices and compliance [10].

In another study, Horowitz, Rein, and Leventhal [11] conducted semi-structured interviews with 19 patients suffering from congestive heart failure (CHF). Most of the patients conceptualized CHF as an acute rather than a chronic disease. They tended to think of their symptoms as problems that could be addressed with treatment. The patients did not seem to recognize that the symptoms were expected to worsen over time. The interviews indicated that patients often sought acute care in emergency rooms when they had exacerbations of their symptoms. They tended not to manage their symptoms on a routine basis as is advised for patients with CHF. The acute disease mental model common among CHF patients may have led them to treat their chronic disease as if it was acute. They should have been using self care on a chronic basis, not just when they had symptoms.

Statistics and Mental Models

Statistical information reported in the media may have a substantial impact on mental models. Interpreting the results of large clinical studies can be very difficult. We often read newspaper articles about astounding results in new clinical studies. These studies lead to the expectation of a large benefit from intervention. The Physicians' Health Study is one example. In this experiment, approximately 22,000 physicians were divided into two groups [12]. One group was assigned to take 325 mg of aspirin every other day. The other half took placebos. The study was stopped early because the benefit was so strong. Those taking aspirin experienced a 72-percent reduction in the rate of myocardial infarction (MI or heart attack). There is little ambiguity. Everyone should take aspirin. Or should they?

The Physicians' Health Study raises a number of important questions. Where does the 72 percent come from? Does it mean that 80 percent of participants would have experienced a heart attack and the percentage was reduced to 8 percent? Well, not exactly. The 72-percent reduction is what epidemiologists refer to as "relative risk reduction." Relative risk reduction is defined by the event rate in the control group minus the event rate in the experimental group divided by the event rate in the control group (see Table 3.1). In the Physicians' Health Study, there were 18 fatal heart attacks in the control group and 5 fatal heart attacks in the experimental group [13]. The calculations are shown in Table 3.2.

Clinical epidemiologists argue that patients should also be given information about the absolute risk reduction (ARR). ARR is simply the event rate in the control group minus the event rate in the experimental group. In the Physicians'

Table 3.1 Calculation of relative risk reduction

$$\frac{CER - EER}{CER}$$

where CER = control event rate
         EER = experimental event rate

Table 3.2 Calculation of absolute risk reduction

- 22,000 participants, half assigned to 325 mg aspirin every other day half to placebo
- 5 fatal MI cases on aspirin, 18 on placebo
- $RRR = (18/11{,}000 - 5/11{,}000)/(18/11{,}000) = 0.72$

Note: Values have been rounded to the second decimal.

Table 3.3 Calculation of absolute risk reduction (ARR) (Permission not needed)

• Simply subtract the absolute risks
ARR = (CER − EER)
Physicians Health
ARR = 18/11,000–5/11,000 = 0.001636 − 0.000454 = 0.001182

Health Study, fatal heart attacks were quite rare in both groups. The event rate in the control group was 18/11,000 while the event rate in the group taking aspirin was 5/11,000. The calculations are in Table 3.3. Less than 0.16 percent (16 percent of a single percentage point) had heart attacks in either group. By taking aspirin every other day, the physicians reduced their chances of dying from a heart attack by approximately 0.4 percent (or about four-tenths of 1 percent). Certainly this looks and feels much less impressive that a "72 percent reduction."

To make things even more complicated, aspirin did not change the life expectancy of the participants. At the end of the first phase of the study, 44 physicians who had taken aspirin had died and 44 physicians who had taken a placebo had died. There was absolutely no difference in the chances of being alive. This is shown in Fig. 3.1. Although the causes of death were slightly different, the total number of deaths summed to the same number. Figure 3.2 shows cardiovascular deaths and nonvascular deaths versus those participants in the study who were alive and healthy at the follow-up. In the figure, all causes of mortality are graphically compressed toward the bottom, indicating that the vast majority of the participants (about 99.6 percent in each group) were alive when the results were published.

Another example of how relative risks are sometimes misconstrued can be seen in the Helsinki Heart Study. In this experimental trial, 2,051 men were

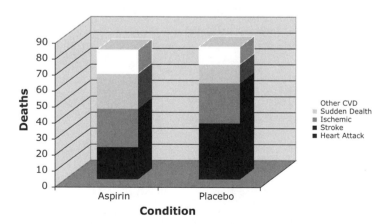

Fig. 3.1 Total mortality in the Aspirin component of the Physicians' Health Study. Overall the number of physicians who died was identical in the Aspirin and the Placebo conditions (Steering Committee of the physicians' Health Study Research Group [12])

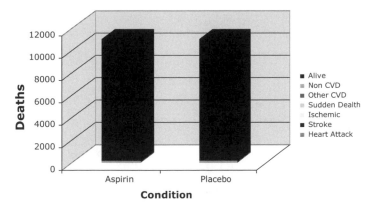

Fig. 3.2 Absolute change in death in the Aspirin component of the Physicians' Health Study. The open area of each column shows the proportion of physicians who were alive and well at the end of the study—approximately 99.6% in both groups

randomly assigned to take Genfibrozil twice daily for 6 years [14]. Genfibrozil is a drug that lowers cholesterol. Another 2,030 men were randomly assigned to take placebos for the same period of time. There were 14 deaths from heart disease in the Genfibrozil group and 19 in the placebo group [15].

Table 3.4 summarizes the calculation of relative risk reduction and the ARR. As reported in the newspapers, there was a 27-percent reduction in relative risk. However, the ARR was about 0.3 percent (three-tenths of 1 percent). This was because virtually everybody in the study was well and free of heart disease at the end of the trial. The 27-percent reduction in deaths from heart disease seems like a substantial benefit. To me as an individual, however, chances of avoiding a heart-attack change by far less than 1 percent. As in the Physicians' Health Study, the Helsinki Heart Study also had a complicated result for total mortality. At the end of the study, 45 participants in the Genfibrozil group had died (2.19 percent of the participants), in comparison with 42 deaths in the placebo group (2.07 percent of the participants). In other words, chances of being alive were slightly better for those taking the placebo, although the difference was not statistically significant (see Fig. 3.3)

When results are reported in terms of relative risk reduction, patients may think that there are enormous benefits associated with popular treatments. This is clearly so with regard to taking cholesterol-reducing medication. Most patients taking these medications think that they are likely to die if they avoid the medication and that the medication provides very strong protection. After all, newspaper articles have informed them that their chances of dying will be

Table 3.4 Calculation of relative risk reduction and absolute risk reduction in the Helsinki Heart Study

- RRR $= (19/2030) - (14/2051)/(19/2030) = 0.27$
- ARR $= 0.0094 - 0.0068 = 0.0025$

Note: figures have been rounded

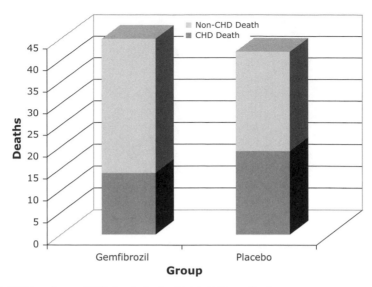

Fig. 3.3 CHD and non-CHD deaths in the Helsinki Heart Study

reduced by 27, 35, or 44 percent. However, at the individual level, chances of dying or having a heart-attack change very modestly. In many cases, the differences in mortality between treated and untreated patients are less than 1 percent. In the case of the Helsinki Heart Study, the chances of being alive for these high-risk men were 98.8 percent in the Gemfibrozil group and 98.9 percent in the Placebo group. These are hardly numbers that would motivate most of us to ask for a prescription. The numbers chosen to describe the benefits of treatment can make a big difference in what patients ask for and what doctors prescribe.

How did so many people develop such high expectations of benefit? One reason is that they were led there by some highly credible sources. Websites from the American Heart Association, pharmaceutical companies and health-care advocates present the risks of heart disease as binary: if you have an elevated risk factor, then you are more likely to have a heart attack. They provide surprisingly little information on how much absolute and relative risk is associated with various factors. As a result, many people have a mental model leading them to believe that a minor elevation in the risk factor makes them very likely to experience a bad outcome. In fact, for most people, minor elevations of a single risk factor have an extremely modest effect on their relative risks of a bad outcome. Furthermore, the mental models associated with treatment often lead people to believe that taking medication alleviates their risks. As we have seen in two examples, the chances of having a bad outcome are changed by a remarkably small amount if medication is taken.

In order to help people understand these issues, clinical epidemiologists have proposed terms such as the number needed to treat (NNT). The NNT is defined as the number of people who would need to be treated in order for one person to be helped. The NNT is simply 1 divided by the absolute risk ratio. In the Physicians' Health Study, for example, the ARR was 0.00118. That was obtained using the calculations shown in Table 3.3 (ARR = 18/11,000 − 5/11,000 = 0.001636 − 0.000454 = 0.001182). In order to calculate the NNT, we simply divide 1 by that number. The result is 846. It is obtained as: 1/0.00118 = 847. This means for each 847 physicians treated with aspirin, one heart attack will be avoided. For the other 846 physicians who take aspirin every other day, no benefit is obtained. The result sounds quite different from the 72-percent reduction in heart attacks noted in the original newspaper articles.

We often act on the basis of our conceptual mental models of illness, and sometimes these models are physiological—they represent our understanding of what is wrong with us. But there are also mental models associated with the probability of *benefit* from treatment. Much of the information about health-care available in the media leads us to believe we will get substantial benefits from preventive treatments. Usually, this is because the information is presented in terms of relative risk reduction. To an individual, relative risk reduction may provide relatively little information. Most people want to know how their own chances of a bad outcome are changed by treatment. In some cases, these chances are changed only very slightly. The point is that there is a lot of information that stimulates incorrect mental models about the expected benefits of treatment. In some of the remaining chapters, we explore these issues in more detail and comment on how they ultimately affect major decisions—societal as well as personal—about health and healthcare.

Mental Models and the People We Most Trust

Understanding risks and health benefits can be pretty complicated. The problems themselves are hard to understand, and there we are constantly confronted with conflicting information. This chapter offers examples of how information about screening can be spun in very different ways. Confronted with such complex and confusing information, many turn to those they trust most. These include nonprofit organizations and trusted public figures. Although most of the public nonprofits are excellent organizations, they have a vested interest in finding cases of the diseases they care about. More cases mean more donations, more research dollars, and a bigger political constituency.

The American Heart Association devotes the entire month of September to cholesterol. They call it "National Cholesterol Awareness Month." Their website tells readers that over 100 million Americans have cholesterol levels that may require treatment. The site links the reader to an industry-sponsored section on cholesterol-lowering drugs, which are described as very effective.

Most of the pharmaceutical companies have eloquent and attractive websites describing their products. The website from Pfizer Pharmaceuticals begins by saying, "We are talking a lot about cholesterol, and high cholesterol levels, but many people don't really understand what it is." The site goes on to explain that LDL cholesterol can lead to heart disease and cites the American Heart Association as saying, "Experts recommend that all adults over the age of 20 should have their cholesterol measured at least once every 5 years." The site emphasizes the need for everybody to be tested and to use the Pfizer product (LIPITOR) if their cholesterol level is elevated. This is good business for Pfizer because, according to their evidence, about one in two adults will qualify for treatment.

The American Cancer Society also emphasizes screening and early detection. Their website recommends a variety of screening tests. For example, the American Cancer Society recommends screening for breast cancer starting at age 40, and clinical breast exams starting at age 20. These recommendations conflict with virtually all scientific organizations that have reviewed the same evidence. The US Preventive Service task force is an independent panel of experts in primary care and prevention that systematically reviews the evidence of effectiveness and develops recommendations for clinical preventive services. They recommend beginning mammography screening at age 50. Similarly, there have been a variety of reviews in other countries, and virtually all of them have concluded that screening is of little value before age 50. The American Cancer Society also states that, beginning at age 50, the PSA blood test and digital rectal exam should be offered each year for all men. Furthermore, they recommend that these tests be done earlier for African American men and men with a family history of prostate cancer.

Both the American Cancer Society and the American Heart Association state that early intervention saves lives. However, it is celebrities rather than physicians and scientists who most often promote these views to the general public. The American Heart Association has a direct link to the Pfizer web page. Pfizer sponsors the "Cholesterol Low-down," a national education program. Actor Henry Winkler promotes the program. Mr. Winkler urges all Americans to get their cholesterol checked in order to "take action today for a healthier heart tomorrow." The stated purpose of Mr. Winkler's advocacy is to "dispel myths about heart disease," and he refers to new "heartbreaking" statistics. According to the website, a 10-percent reduction in cholesterol might reduce the incidence of heart disease by 30 percent. (We will return to these numbers in a full discussion of lower cholesterol in Chapter 7.) Before Henry Winkler's role as the national spokesman, Regis Philbin, Debbie Allen, Dick Clark, Mary Wilson, Vicki Lawrence, and Valerie Harper had held the role.

One study examined the impact of celebrity endorsements on screening for breast cancer, prostate cancer, and colorectal cancer: 360 women aged 40 and older and 140 men aged 50 and older participated in a national survey. The survey used a random digit-dialing method to ensure representativeness. Nearly three-quarters of the women respondents reported having seen or heard a celebrity talk about mammography, 63 percent of the men had heard of celebrity endorsements for PSA testing, and about half of the adults had heard celebrity endorsements for colorectal cancer screening. Figure 3.4 summarizes

Fig. 3.4 Effects of celebrity endorsements for cancer screening. (Larson et al., [16])

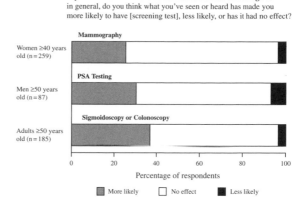

the impact of celebrity endorsements on people old enough to be tested. About one-quarter of the women who had heard celebrities endorse mammography reported being more likely to get the test. Similarly, 31 percent of the men reported that they were more likely to get the PSA test because they had heard a celebrity endorsement. For colorectal cancer screening, 37 percent of the respondents reported being more likely to get an invasive test because of a celebrity endorsement [16].

This chapter has challenged two common beliefs about the nature of illness. First, we challenged the belief that components of the body work in a linear fashion. Certainly few physicians or physiologists would argue for a linear model. Nevertheless, the belief in the linearity of biological systems is commonly promoted to support treatments for common chronic illnesses. The acute disease model is the second concept challenged in this chapter. Our healthcare system, and many of our beliefs about the potential of healthcare, is based on the premise that disease can be found and fixed. Again, it would be hard to find a medical professional who would not recognize that most of the cost and effort in contemporary healthcare is devoted to chronic disease. However, how is the potential of medicine to deal with chronic disease communicated to the public? Most of the public nonprofit charities cling to the message that common chronic diseases can be found and fixed.

We have perpetuated some questionable beliefs about health and about the care people must receive for chronic medical problems. The consequence is excessive cost in the chase for treatments that may be of limited value. The following chapters spell out some of the reasons why we are being led in the wrong direction and suggest some new mental models for shaping our choices. In health and healthcare, these models require continual evaluation, and healthcare professionals and researchers are accustomed to this reevaluation process. Over the course of time, few approaches to medical care remain constant, and consumers as well as healthcare providers will have to learn how and why our policies and practices will change.

References

1. Turner RB, Bauer R, Woelkart K, Hulsey TC, Gangemi JD. An evaluation of Echinacea angustifolia in experimental rhinovirus infections. *N Engl J Med.* Jul 28 2005; 353(4):341–348.
2. Ackoff R. *The Democratic Corporation.* New York: Oxford University Press; 1994.
3. Checkland P. Systems theory and management thinking. *Am Behav Sci.* 1994;38(1): 75–91.
4. Gharajedaghi J AR. Mechanisms, organisms, and social systems. *Strateg Manag J.* 1984; 5: 289–300.
5. Holman H, Lorig K. Patients as partners in managing chronic disease. Partnership is a prerequisite for effective and efficient health care [editorial; comment]. *BMJ (Clinical Research Ed.).* 2000;320(7234):526–527.
6. Ware JE, Jr., Bayliss MS, Rogers WH, Kosinski M, Tarlov AR. Differences in 4-year health outcomes for elderly and poor, chronically ill patients treated in HMO and fee-for-service systems. Results from the Medical Outcomes Study [see comments]. *JAMA.* 1996;276(13):1039–1047.
7. Kaplan RM. Two pathways to prevention. *Am Psychol.* 2000;55(4):382–396.
8. Kaplan RM. The Ziggy theorem: toward an outcomes-focused health psychology. *Health Psychol.* 1994;13(6):451–460.
9. McGinnis JM, Foege WH. Actual causes of death in the United States [see comments]. *JAMA.* 1993;270(18):2207–2212.
10. Rabin C, Leventhal H, Goodin S. Conceptualization of disease timeline predicts post-treatment distress in breast cancer patients. *Health Psychol.* Jul 2004;23(4):407–412.
11. Horowitz CR, Rein SB, Leventhal H. A story of maladies, misconceptions and mishaps: effective management of heart failure. *Soc Sci Med.* Feb 2004;58(3):631–643.
12. Steering Committee of the Physicians' Health Study Research Group. Final report on the aspirin component of the ongoing Physicians' Health Study. *N Engl J Med.* Jul 20 1989;321(3):129–135.
13. Findings from the aspirin component of the ongoing Physicians' Health Study. *N Engl J Med.* Jan 28 1988;318(4):262–264.
14. Huttunen JK, Manninen V, Manttari M, et al. The Helsinki Heart Study: central findings and clinical implications. *Ann Med.* Apr 1991;23(2):155–159.
15. Frick MH, Elo O, Haapa K, et al. Helsinki Heart Study: primary-prevention trial with gemfibrozil in middle-aged men with dyslipidemia. Safety of treatment, changes in risk factors, and incidence of coronary heart disease. *N Engl J Med.* Nov 12 1987;317(20): 1237–1245.
16. Larson RJ, Woloshin S, Schwartz LM, Welch HG. Celebrity endorsements of cancer screening. *J Natl Cancer Inst.* May 4 2005;97(9):693–695.

Chapter 4
What Is Disease and When Does It Begin?

A close friend recently shared her reaction to being diagnosed with cancer. The diagnosis occurred 11 years ago, but her memories are vivid. "I can remember the day my doctor told me I had cancer," she said. "That was the day my life changed. Before that, I had been completely healthy."

My friend talked as though her cancer began the day her doctor told her about it. But is that really when the disease started? Most likely, the disease had been developing for years before the diagnosis. In this chapter, we will explore a variety of misperceptions about chronic disease. These misperceptions of chronic illness are common and may have a profound effect on how we make decisions about treatment, how resources in healthcare are spent, and why we often neglect to look in the right place for resolutions to health problems.

Common Perceptions of Chronic Disease

Beliefs about chronic illness influence decisions about screening, treatment, and health habits. A variety of common beliefs about the origin of a disease may not be correct. For example, many people think that disease starts near the time of diagnosis. However, evidence suggests that many chronic diseases start years before they are diagnosed [1, 2]. A second common belief is that diseases are binary—you either have the disease or you do not have it. In reality, most chronic diseases exist on some kind of continuum. A third common belief is that all diseases must be treated and that untreated disease will likely lead to death or disability. In fact, diseases have natural histories. Sometimes they get better on their own. In other cases, chronic diseases linger but never have an important impact on a person or his or her lifestyle. Finally, it is commonly believed that bad health outcomes usually result from failure to detect disease early. Certainly this is true in some cases. Yet, in other cases early detection is of little value. For example, early detection of a disease that will not eventually result in death, disability, or symptoms maybe of little importance [3]. Similarly, detection of a disease for which there is no effective treatment cannot lead to a remedy that will make the patient better.

R.M. Kaplan, *Disease, Diagnoses, and Dollars*, DOI 10.1007/978-0-387-74045-4_4,
© Springer Science+Business Media, LLC 2009

More Is More, But Is More Better?

Melanoma is the most deadly form of skin cancer. It would seem a good idea to find more cases of melanoma and to find them as early in the disease process as possible. However, at least in older adults, the benefits of early detection of melanoma may not be so clear. Welch and colleagues [4] studied US Medicare records between 1986 and 2001. They noted a significant increase in the incidence of melanoma during this period. Furthermore, they discovered there was a parallel increase in early-stage cases. However, the rate of diagnosis for late-stage disease and the mortality from melanoma did not change at all during this interval (Fig. 4.1).

Why was the rate of melanoma diagnosis increasing? Welch and colleagues argued that there is a reservoir of undiagnosed mild melanoma. These cases, particularly in elderly Medicare patients, are not likely to reduce life expectancy.

However, an increased rate of biopsy could reasonably be expected to yield more diagnosed cases. Indeed, this is what the researchers found. For each of 14 years, the researchers estimated the rate of skin biopsy for the nine areas of the USA that report data to the National Cancer Institute's Surveillance Epidemiology and End Results (SEER) program. Data from the SEER program also allowed them to estimate the rate of discovery for new cases of cancer. There was an observation for each of the nine geographic locations for each of the 14 years, resulting in the 126 data points shown in Fig. 4.2. The graph shows that the more we look, the more we find. New cases of melanoma are systematically related to the use of more biopsies. Welch and colleagues suggest that many of the biopsies done for older people offer little clinical benefit. As shown in Fig. 4.1, finding more cases does not result in a reduced melanoma death rate. Among the newly diagnosed cases, many will receive treatment even though the treatment is not likely to extend life or improve quality of life [4]. Of course, this study has important limitations. It could be that there are more biopsies because there is truly more cancer and that treatment is saving those who have the

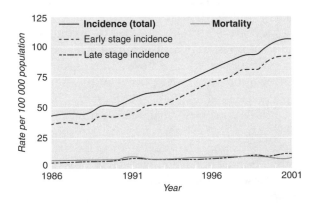

Fig. 4.1 Incidence of melanoma and death from melanoma between 1986 and 2001. (Welch et al. [4])

Fig. 4.2 Skin biopsies and melanoma 100,000/ population in 1986, 2001, and the interval 1987–2000. (Welch et al. [4])

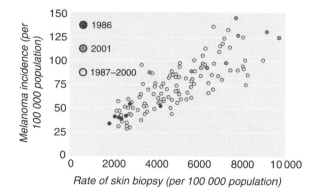

diagnosis. Only more research will allow us to evaluate this alternative. However, Welch and colleagues make a very persuasive case that more aggressive testing results in more aggressive treatment, but more treatment does not leave people much better off.

Prostate cancer offers another example of diagnosis that adds to the caseload, but does not increase life expectancy. For many years, urologists have reported a strong correlation between age and positive biopsy for prostate cancer, and it has even been suggested that all men will develop prostate cancer if they live long enough. A study of accidental deaths in Detroit men shows a systematic relationship between prostate cancer and age. Of those routinely autopsied, only about 1 in 12 men have prostate cancer if they died in their 20 s, but the proportion increases to 8 of 10 men by age 80, as shown in Fig. 4.3. (Note in the figure, the relationship between age and prostate cancer is the same for both Caucasian and African-American men.) Thomas Stamey, a Stanford professor of urology, reported that his institution performed biopsies of every prostate that had been removed beginning in 1983. They also had data on PSA tests. Stamey reported that prostate cancer rates systematically increase as men get older, but that the PSA test related only to prostate size, not to prostate cancer. Although Stamey had been a major advocate for the PSA test in the 1980 s, by 2004 he published an article declaring, "The era of serum prostate specific antigen as a marker for biopsy of the prostate and detecting prostate cancer is now over in the USA [6]."

Fig. 4.3 Prostate cancer among 525 Detroit men who died of violence or in accidents; 314 African Americans (dark bars), and 211 Caucasians (light bars). (Sakr et al. [5])

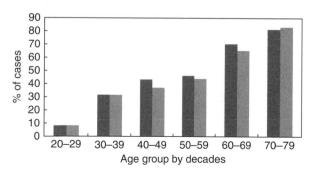

When Does Chronic Disease Begin?

The day of diagnosis is an important milestone. Being told you have a chronic illness is very scary, and for many people it is life-changing. Yet, date of diagnosis is rarely the date that the disease started. In many cases the two dates are not even close.

Figure 4.4 summarizes the atherosclerosis timeline, illustrated with a kind of "time lapse" artist's conception of how a section of coronary artery can deteriorate over time. Over the course of a lifetime, plaque builds up under the endothelial wall of the artery, and the artery gradually narrows. Eventually, this plaque can rupture, resulting in a blood clot that may completely close the coronary artery. This is called a myocardial infarction (MI) or heart attack.

Many people think their disease started the day of their heart attack. However, Fig. 4.4 summarizes anatomical evidence that the process takes decades. Foam cells may become abnormal in the first decade of life. By the mid-20s, fatty streaks begin to develop within the artery. From the third decade of life many people develop intermediate lesions, and the narrowing of the artery continues. By the fourth decade, many people have fibrous plaque and damage to smooth muscle and collagen. Ultimately, the heart attack is a result of a gradual process that has been evolving over the course of at least four decades [8].

There is ample evidence to support this view. Some of the first studies involved veterans from foreign wars. In 1955, Enos and colleagues reported on 300 autopsies from people who had died in the Korean conflict [9]. The average age at death was 22.1 years. Among these young men, 77.3 percent had

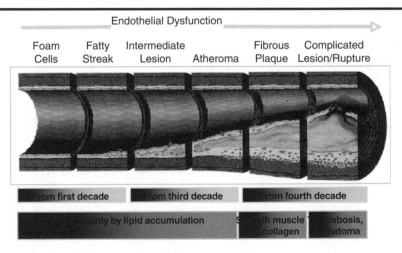

Stary et al. *Circulation.* 1995;92:1355–1374.

Fig. 4.4 Atherosclerosis timeline. (Adapted from Pepine et al. [7])

early signs of coronary artery disease. In 1971, McNamara and colleagues reported on autopsies of 105 Vietnam casualties of [8] the same average age—22.1 years [10]. They found that 45 percent had evidence of significant coronary artery disease. Figure 4.5 summarizes the findings from a series of autopsies by Strong and colleagues [11]. They examined the abdominal aortas of 2,876 young people who had died of violent causes in the USA. These deaths include traffic accidents, murders, and suicides, but none were deaths from known disease. The innermost part of an artery is called the intima and the investigators looked at the percentage of the intima affected by disease. Although the young victims were more than two and a half times more likely to be male, the group included both black and while and both male and female victims. The top two lines in the figure summarize the proportion young people in the 15- to 19-year-old age group who had lesions that were greater than 5 percent of the intimal surface. Remarkably, nearly 90 percent of subjects had these lesions. By age 30, 95 percent of the young people had these lesions. Raised lesions might be cause for genuine clinical concern. The figure shows that by age 30, fully 40 percent of these young victims had raised lesions.

While the indications of what constitutes coronary artery disease were different in the studies by Enos, McNamara, and Strong, all three of the studies lead to one inescapable conclusion: Even among very young men, the incidence of early signs of coronary artery disease is stunningly high. The reservoir of undiagnosed coronary disease is huge. Other studies have come to the same conclusion [12, 13] using different methodology including noninvasive imaging of the coronary arteries [13]. Each shows essentially the same result. If we look for disease even early in life, it is likely to be found.

Many years ago, Armenian and Lilienfeld [14] reported that cancer may take a very long time to develop. The original hypothesis was published in 1974 [15] and was followed up with a detailed review in 1983 [14]. Among the many

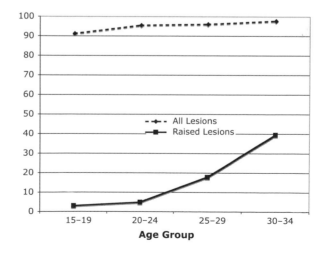

Fig. 4.5 Abdominal aortic lesions > 5% of intimal surface and raised lesions 2876 who died from non-disease causes between the ages 15 and 34 and underwent autopsy. (Adapted from Strong et al. [11])

studies that support this idea are investigations of migration. It has been known for some time that women from southern Italy have a lower rate of breast cancer than women in northern Italy. However, many women migrate from south to north or from north to south. Berrinal and a group of Epidemiologists from Milan studied these migration patterns. They found that the risk of breast cancer is most associated with the place of residence early in childhood. Women who migrated from the south to the north before puberty still maintained the low characteristic risk pattern of southern Italians. This may suggest that the incubation period for breast cancer may be 20 years and could be as long as 40 years. The date of the diagnosis tells much more about the time someone suspected the disease than it does about the date the disease began.

Other studies have examined the relationship between cigarette smoking and breast cancer. Studies have shown that the amount of exposure to tobacco is related to the development of several cancers. One analysis of nearly 90,000 female participants in a Canadian study about breast cancer found that having started smoking early in life was one of the best predictors of breast cancer. After controlling for total exposure to cigarettes, total duration of smoking remained an important predictor. This suggests that exposure to cigarettes early in life is an important risk factor and that the latency period for the development of breast cancer could be many decades [16]. Often, when a chronic disease like cancer or coronary artery disease is discovered, we feel that emergency action must be taken. Having a heart attack is an emergency and it is clear that emergency action is in order. That can save lives. However, the diagnosis of other chronic diseases may be the identification of a process that has been going on for many years. Often the diagnosis does not signal an emergency because it is not clear that the consequences of taking immediate actions outweigh the benefits.

What are the Implications of These Findings?

Diagnosis is the first step on the way to treatment. It is very difficult not to offer a treatment when a disease has been discovered. We know, for example, that a high percentage of all adults have narrowing of their coronary arteries. If tests are used to look inside the arteries, the likely result is that disease will be found. Once disease is discovered, there will be motivation to provide treatment.

Coronary artery bypass graft (CABG) surgery uses harvested arteries or veins from elsewhere in the patient's body to bypass narrowed coronary arteries and improve the blood supply to the heart muscle. It is a very complex procedure that requires opening of the chest, removal of ribs, and the use of a heat and lung machine. Transluminal coronary angioplasty (PTCA) is coronary angioplasty, a procedure in which a catheter is inserted to open up a blocked coronary artery and restore blood flow to the heart muscle. It is less invasive, less expensive, and faster to perform than CABG. The term angioplasty literally means "reshape." A balloon is inserted and inflated to reshape the narrowed artery. Sometimes a device known as a "stent" is placed in the artery to help keep it open.

Using Medicare claims data, Wennberg and colleagues studied the relationship between the use of angiography, a method to look inside the arteries, and the likelihood that people would get invasive treatment for heart disease. They accomplished this by studying Medicare claims from 306 hospital referral agencies in the USA. The result is shown in Fig. 4.6. The population of Medicare claims in the USA (everyone in the USA falls into one of the 306 services areas) they discovered a systematic relationship between the incidence of angiography following a heart attack and the likelihood of intervention. Each dot in the figure represents one of the 306 hospital service areas. The slope of the line suggests that there is approximately one intervention, either by surgery or by angioplasty, for each 1.5 episodes of angiography. Further study, however, revealed essentially no correlation between the number of procedures and the prevalence of disease.

Acute MI is the most common cause of morbidity and mortality in both the USA and Canada. However, the two countries approach the treatment of cardiovascular disease (CVD) differently. Invasive cardiac procedures such as coronary angiography are performed considerably more often in the USA than in Canada. Some years ago, my colleagues at UCSD noted that about 8 of every 10 well-insured patients in San Diego received angiography following a heart attack if they were treated in private hospitals [17]. However, only 40 percent patients at the San Diego Veterans Affairs Health Center received the procedure following a heart attack. In Vancouver, only 20 percent of post-MI patients got angiography, and only 10 percent of patients in Sweden received the procedure. This variation might be acceptable to the doctors and well-insured patients in San Diego if we knew that more care led to better health. However, there was little evidence that more aggressive care produced better results. Controlling for the seriousness of the heart attack (measured by and index of how well the heart is able to pump blood), the probability of surviving an MI in San Diego, Vancouver, and Sweden was comparable.

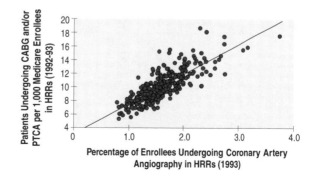

Fig. 4.6 Relationship between angiography and procedures in Medicare claims. (Dartmouth Atlas of Health Care, 1998 [18])

One study evaluated the use of invasive of cardiac procedures in the USA and Canada by comparing the care of 224,258 elderly Medicare recipients in the USA and 9,444 older patients in Ontario, Canada. Each of these patients had been the victim of heart attack after 1991. Among American patients, 34.9 percent underwent coronary angiography, while only 6.7 percent of the Canadian patients received this procedure (see Fig. 4.7). Having coronary angiography increases the likelihood that other invasive procedures will be performed. Among the American patients, 11.7 percent underwent transluminal coronary angioplasty in comparison with 1.5 percent of the Canadian patients. Furthermore, 10.6 percent of the American patients vs. only 1.4 percent of the Canadian patients underwent coronary artery bypass surgery (Fig. 4.8). Figure 4.9 summarizes the mortality rates for these patients. It might be presumed that American patients are better off because they are more likely to obtain the latest and more "aggressive" procedures. However, mortality rates 30 days following the attack were comparable in the two countries (21.4 percent vs. 22.3 percent). Furthermore, the mortality rates 1 year later were virtually identical (34.3 percent in the

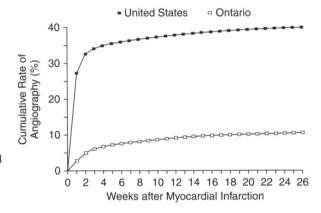

Fig. 4.7 Cumulative rate of angiography in the USA and Canada by weeks following myocardial infarction. (From Tu et al. [19])

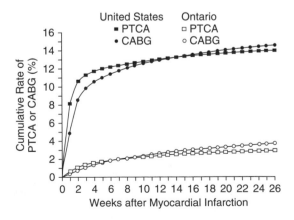

Fig. 4.8 Cumulative rate of PT and Coronary Artery Bypass Graft (CABG) surgery in the USA and Canada by weeks following myocardial infarction. (From Tu et al. [19])

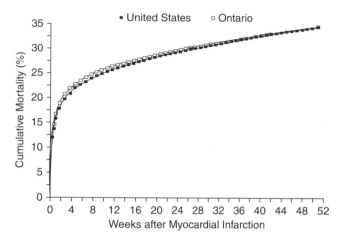

Fig. 4.9 Cumulative mortality in the USA and Canada by weeks following Myocardial Infarction. (From Tu et al. [19])

USA vs. 34.4 percent in Canada). These data suggest that the use of high-technology medical procedures is much more likely in the American system than in the Canadian healthcare system. However, there is no clear evidence that patients benefit, at least in terms of survival [19].

These results are challenging. They suggest that more may not be better. Countries that look harder for disease find more disease. This is exactly what we would expect if the disease-reservoir hypothesis is correct. On the other hand, finding more disease is clearly related to treating more disease. The difficulty is that countries that treat more do not necessarily have better patient outcomes. In fact, some evidence suggests that more aggressive care results in poorer rather than better patient outcomes [20, 21].

A second implication is that screening may not always be valuable. Arguments against screening have been most clearly articulated in a book by Gilbert Welch [22]. Welch, a practicing physician, knows how difficult it is to deliver a diagnosis of cancer. On the other hand, he systematically demonstrates that not all cancer results in poor outcomes. Some cancers do not progress, and there is even some evidence that untreated cancers can be conquered by a well-functioning immune system. Unfortunately, we know very little about the natural history of cancer because the disease is rarely left untreated. We do know that the value of screening for cancer can be somewhat limited. Because this is such a complex and controversial problem, an entire chapter (Chapter 5) is devoted to it. Suffice it to say here that we still have relatively little evidence that cancer screening is a good use of resources [23]. We do know that screening is typically quite expensive and that the cost of screening is quite high in relation to other uses of healthcare resources. Cost-effectiveness analysis is complex and controversial, so an entire chapter (Chapter 9) is devoted to this problem as well.

Primary versus Secondary Prevention

This chapter has raised some thorny issues. It began by challenging the commonly held belief that disease starts near the time of diagnosis. Although this may be true for acute diseases, most chronic diseases develop slowly, over the course of many years. By the time they are diagnosed, it is likely that the disease has been evolving gradually. And it remained unknown only because diagnostic technology had not discovered it. Sometimes the disease went undiagnosed because the patient lived in an area where doctors did not perform the test or because the doctors did not use tests powerful enough to find the problem. For example, the smallest prostate cancer that can be detected with modern tests is a mass of at least 1 billion cells. That same tumor, at one point, had only 1 million cells, and before that 100,000. We only call it disease when it reaches the point where modern technology can find it. This challenges the common belief that disease is binary. In other words, it may not be appropriate to think of diseases as either present or absent. Most disease falls somewhere along a continuum.

We also challenged the belief that all diseases must be treated. In fact, most of us have multiple problems and these problems may not affect us during our lifetimes. Of course, this makes the decision about how to care for ourselves and what medical services to use much more complex. Early detection of disease may result in better health outcomes, but there are also circumstances in which early detection may do no good, or even cause harm. In Chapter 5, we will deal with methods that help sort out this complex set of problems.

Perhaps the most challenging lesson is that most of what we call preventive medicine is really not about preventing disease. Screening tests are used to detect diseases that are already progressing. The art and science we call "preventive medicine" is often about early detection rather than disease prevention. The evidence reviewed in this chapter suggests that much of what we believe to be "early" detection is really detection of disease at a relatively advanced phase.

There is evidence that some things really do prevent disease. For example, cigarette smoking is clearly related to the development of cancer and heart disease. By preventing young people from smoking, we could significantly reduce the burden of these terrible diseases. However, we devote remarkably little attention and effort to true prevention. The US Centers for Disease Control and the National Institutes of Health (NIH) have developed a National action plan for the prevention and treatment of heart disease. Part of the challenge is that 95 cents of each dollar spent on heart disease and stroke care in the USA is devoted to treatment, and only about 5 cents per dollar is devoted to prevention [24]. Certainly we can do better.

References

1. Black WC. Overdiagnosis: an underrecognized cause of confusion and harm in cancer screening. *J Natl Cancer Inst*.Aug 16 2000;92(16):1280–1282.

2. Welch HG, Black WC. Using autopsy series to estimate the disease "reservoir" for ductal carcinoma in situ of the breast: how much more breast cancer can we find? *Ann Intern Med.*1997;127(11):1023–1028.

3. Black WC, Welch HG. Screening for disease. *AJR Am J Roentgenol.*1997;168(1):3–11.

4. Welch HG, Woloshin S, Schwartz LM. Skin biopsy rates and incidence of melanoma: population based ecological study. *BMJ.*Sep 3 2005;331(7515):481.

5. Sakr WA, Grignon DJ, Haas GP, Heilbrun LK, Pontes JE, Crissman JD. Age and racial distribution of prostatic intraepithelial neoplasia. *Eur Urol.*1996;30(2): 138–144.

6. Stamey TA, Caldwell M, McNeal JE, Nolley R, Hemenez M, Downs J. The prostate specific antigen era in the United States is over for prostate cancer: what happened in the last 20 years? *J Urol.*Oct 2004;172(4 Pt 1):1297–1301.

7. Pepine CJ, et al. *A definition of advanced types of atherosclerotic lesions and a histological classification of atherosclerosis.* Am. J. Cardiol. 1998; 82:10 (Supplement): 235–278.

8. Stary HC, Chandler AB, Dinsmore RE, et al. A definition of advanced types of atherosclerotic lesions and a histological classification of atherosclerosis. A report from the Committee on Vascular Lesions of the Council on Arteriosclerosis, American Heart Association. *Circulation.*Sep 1 1995;92(5):1355–1374.

9. Enos WF, Jr., Beyer JC, Holmes RH. Pathogenesis of coronary disease in American soldiers killed in Korea. *J Am Med Assoc.*Jul 16 1955;158(11):912–914.

10. McNamara JJ, Molot MA, Stremple JF, Cutting RT. Coronary artery disease in combat casualties in Vietnam. *JAMA.*May 17 1971;216(7):1185–1187.

11. Strong JP, Malcom GT, McMahan CA, et al. Prevalence and extent of atherosclerosis in adolescents and young adults: implications for prevention from the Pathobiological Determinants of Atherosclerosis in Youth Study. *JAMA.*Feb 24 1999;281(8):727–735.

12. McGill HC, Jr., McMahan CA, Zieske AW, et al. Association of Coronary Heart Disease Risk Factors with microscopic qualities of coronary atherosclerosis in youth. *Circulation.* Jul 25 2000;102(4):374–379.

13. Tuzcu EM, Kapadia SR, Tutar E, et al. High prevalence of coronary atherosclerosis in asymptomatic teenagers and young adults: evidence from intravascular ultrasound. *Circulation.*Jun 5 2001;103(22):2705–2710.

14. Armenian HK, Lilienfeld AM. Incubation period of disease. *Epidemiol Rev.*1983;5:1–15.

15. Armenian HK, Lilienfeld AM. The distribution of incubation periods of neoplastic diseases. *Am J Epidemiol.*Feb 1974;99(2):92–100.

16. Terry PD, Miller AB, Rohan TE. Cigarette smoking and breast cancer risk: a long latency period? *Int J Cancer.*Aug 20 2002;100(6):723–728.

17. Nicod P, Gilpin EA, Dittrich H, et al. Trends in use of coronary angiography in subacute phase of myocardial infarction. *Circulation.*Sep 1991;84(3):1004–1015.

18. Wennberg JE. *The Dartmouth Atlas of Health Care in the United States.* Hanover, NH: Trustees of Dartmouth College; 1998.

19. Tu JV, Pashos CL, Naylor CD, et al. Use of cardiac procedures and outcomes in elderly patients with myocardial infarction in the United States and Canada. *N Engl J Med.*May 22 1997;336(21):1500–1505.

20. Fisher ES, Wennberg DE, Stukel TA, Gottlieb DJ, Lucas FL, Pinder EL. The implications of regional variations in Medicare spending. Part 2: health outcomes and satisfaction with care. *Ann Intern Med.*Feb 18 2003;138(4):288–298.

21. Fisher ES, Wennberg DE, Stukel TA, Gottlieb DJ, Lucas FL, Pinder EL. The implications of regional variations in Medicare spending. Part 1: the content, quality, and accessibility of care. *Ann Intern Med.*Feb 18 2003;138(4):273–287.

22. Welch HG. *Should I Be Tested for Cancer?* Berkeley, CA: University of California Press; 2004.

23. Kaplan RM. Screening for cancer: are resources being used wisely? *Recent Results Cancer Res*.2005;166:315–334.
24. Mosca L, Arnett DK, Dracup K, et al. Task force on strategic research direction: population/outcomes/epidemiology/social science subgroup key science topics report. *Circulation*.Nov 12 2002;106(20):e167–172.

Chapter 5
Screening for Cancer

The American Cancer Society has promoted breast cancer screening through a number of celebrities, including Soraya, a Colombian Grammy Award winning singer and songwriter with great appeal in the Hispanic community. Soraya is a 36-year-old breast cancer survivor. She is also a spokeswoman for the Susan G. Komen Breast Cancer Foundation. In 2006, the ACS estimated that 212,920 women in the USA would be diagnosed with breast cancer. Furthermore, the society projected some 40,970 breast cancer deaths for 2006. Stunned by these data, Soraya decided to take a break from her music career to promote mammography, the American Cancer Society's main weapon in the war against the disease.[1] In the official view of the ACS, mammography is the essential tool for identifying cancer early so that it can be stopped in its tracks.

Yet, despite the broad appeal and acceptance of mammography and other cancer-screening tests, there is lingering concern about the scientific justification for their use. The issues are complex and often emotionally charged. In this chapter, we will look into the controversy and consider the impact of screening tests on patients and on healthcare costs.

There are at least three important approaches to tumor prevention. One approach involves interventions to reduce cancer exposures or to manipulate genetic predispositions so that cancer never begins. A second approach requires screening so that disease can be detected and treated early. The third approach involves treatment of established disease to prevent it from progressing further. Among these three approaches, the second—screening for early detection—has received the most support from healthcare professionals and the greatest acceptance by the general public.

The American Cancer Society and other groups around the world have launched intensive campaigns to persuade the public that an aggressive approach to screening and medical intervention saves a significant number of lives. But do the facts bear out these conclusions about screening and medical intervention? The belief that screening saves lives is built on a foundation of

---

[1] *Miami Herald* Mon, Sep. 26, 2005, Singer a voice for breast-cancer victims by Jerry Berrio.

R.M. Kaplan, *Disease, Diagnoses, and Dollars*, DOI 10.1007/978-0-387-74045-4_5,
© Springer Science+Business Media, LLC 2009

conflicting evidence. And more problematically, our faith in screening has resulted in the rapid growth of cancer-screening programs, to the point where they now consume an extremely large share of our healthcare resources, which in turn means that less money is available to spend on other important health-care programs. Ultimately, exaggerated faith in cancer screening may harm public health by absorbing resources that might have been better used else-where. I want to begin looking in detail at this controversial topic by offering documentation of the public enthusiasm for screening.

Public Enthusiasm for Screening

Americans are enthusiastic about cancer screening. In one recent public opinion poll, Schwartz and colleagues interviewed a random sample of 500 adults selected from throughout the USA. Some 87 percent of the respondents reported that cancer screening is almost always a good idea, and most (approxi-mately 74 percent) endorsed the belief that cancer screening saves lives [1]. Moreover, 77 percent of male respondents said they would continue trying to have the PSA test even if their doctor did not recommend it, and 74 percent said that they would continue to have colonoscopy or sigmoidoscopy when it was not recommended [1]. Aronowitz documented the tireless campaign by the American Cancer Society to persuade the public not to delay in obtaining cancer tests. In fact, the campaign was prominent throughout the entire twen-tieth century, despite continuing questions about the efficacy of early detection [2]. Apparently, these messages have been effective. Schwartz and colleagues, in the study cited above, note that only 2 percent of the population feels that there are too many cancer-screening tests.

Let us consider some other examples. Persuasive evidence suggests that pap smears performed on a yearly basis provide almost no information beyond what pap smears done at 3-year intervals provide [3]. However, the survey results suggest that 58 percent of women would try to maintain their current schedule of pap smears even if their doctor recommended more time between tests. Similarly, even though several evidence-based reviews suggest that mam-mography might provide little or no value for women older than age 75 [4, 5], there is very little organized effort, at least in the USA, for establishing a recommended upper age limit for this kind of screening. It should be noted, however, that the USA is in a minority of countries that do not recommend an age at which to stop screening: In Finland, screening ends at age 59, while Australia, Canada, and Iceland stop at age 69. The UK stops at age 64, and Sweden only screens until age 69 [6]. And even in the USA, the rate of screening for older women falls off after the age of about 75, suggesting that physicians intuitively know the diminished value of the test and stop ordering it [7]. Two related questions then face us: Why is there not a widely publicized age-limit recommendation, and what effect would such a recommendation have on the public's perception? (The Schwartz study found that 41 percent of the population would label an 80-year-old who declined a mammogram to be "irresponsible.")

How strong is the belief that more testing is always better than less? It seems the public is not deterred even by bad experiences with tests. Over a third of the men in the Schwartz survey had experienced at least one false positive. Yet, in retrospect, 98 percent of these individuals were glad they had taken the test, and most would do it again. In fact, 100 percent of those who had experienced a false-positive PSA test were still glad that the tests had been administered [1].

The public is clearly persuaded that cancer screening is a good idea. At the same time, professional organizations that have systematically reviewed the evidence have raised serious questions about the benefits of common tests such as mammography (particularly for the pre-menopausal woman) [8] and the PSA test [9–13]. Is the between professionals and consumers serious enough to require a change in public-health policy and education?

Questions about the Value of Screening on Public Health

One of the most challenging studies about the effectiveness of screening comes from data collected in a research project on breast cancer in France [14]. The study found that while in 1980, there were only 300 mammography machines in France, by the year 2000, 2,511mammography machines were being actively used to screen French women. Figure 5.1 shows the increase in the number of cases of breast cancer detected in France during this interval. In 1980, French doctors were diagnosing about 20,000 cases of breast cancer per year. By the year 2000, there were 20,364 more cases diagnosed than had been discovered in 1980. This stunning 100-percent increase in diagnoses over 20 years (1980–2000) should in fact *not* be stunning, but expected if there is a reservoir of undiagnosed cases. However, we would also assume that early detection would result in a decline in the number of women who died from breast cancer, based on the belief that early detection should help large numbers of women survive longer. But the news, unfortunately, is not so good. In the USA, the rate of death from breast cancer has been constant over the last 40 years, despite substantial increases in the number of cases detected. Figure 5.1 shows that the same is so in France. If anything, there has been a slight increase in the number of women who died of breast cancer, even adjusted for population growth. Since the number of diagnoses has gone up, it appears that more women are surviving breast cancer. However, the alternative explanation, derived from the disease-reservoir hypothesis, is that screening has led to the discovery of more cases of nonthreatening breast cancer.

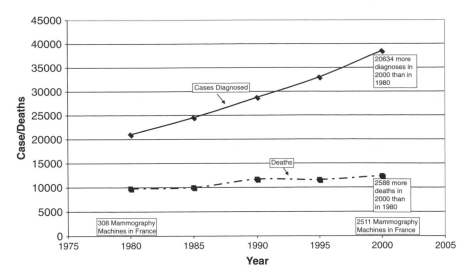

Fig. 5.1 Breast cancer diagnoses and deaths in France: 1980–2000. During that period the number mammography machines increased eight-fold, the number of women diagnoses nearly doubled, but deaths slightly increased rather than decreased as would be expected if more cases were caught early. (Duperray and Junrod [14])

Biases in the Interpretation of Screening Studies

In order to understand controversies and misunderstandings surrounding screening, it is necessary to consider two biases: lead-time bias and length bias.

Lead-Time Bias

Cancer screening may result in early detection of disease. Survival is typically calculated from the date that disease is documented until death. Since screening is associated with earlier disease detection, the interval between detection and death is longer for screened cases than for unscreened cases. Epidemiologists refer to this as *lead-time bias*. Figure 5.2 illustrates this bias.

Imagine that two men developed prostate cancer in 1990 and both died in 2003. Hypothetically, the progression of the cancer was the same in these two men. The man represented by the top line of Fig. 5.2 was screened in 1990 and the cancer was detected. After this diagnosis, he lived 13 additional years, before his death in 2003. The man shown on the lower line did not receive screening but was diagnosed with prostate cancer shortly after he developed urinary symptoms in 2000. After his diagnosis, he lived three additional years. Survival for the man represented at the top appears to be much longer than that for the man represented on the bottom, even though the interval between developing cancer and dying is exactly the same.

Lead Time Bias

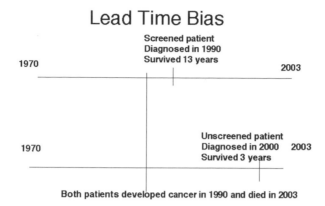

Fig. 5.2 Example of lead-time bias. Two patients get cancer at the same time in 1990 (*vertical line*) and die at the same time in 2003. Both survived the cancer an equal duration of time. However, it appears that the person represented by the top horizontal line survived longer because the disease was detected earlier

Figure 5.2 shows changes in survival among those diagnosed with prostate cancer according to the ACS. These data prompted this conclusion: "Over the past 30 years, the survival rate for all stages combined has increased from 50 percent to 87 percent [15]." The report also concluded that these changes were attributable to advances in cancer diagnosis and treatment.

The claims made by the ACS are doubtful, and have even been dubbed the "myth of 5-year survival [16]." Observational (nonrandomized) studies are unable to separate lead-time bias from treatment effect, and it has been suggested that increased survival associated with screening can be attributed to lead time and not to early detection and treatment [17, 18]. The only way to eliminate lead-time bias is to perform randomized clinical trials with long-term follow-up. In randomized trials, all participants have an equal chance of being assigned to the treatment or to a control group. The reason these trials are important is that the control group is used to learn about the natural history of the disease. In other words, we can determine how many people die of cancer if we do not screen and treat them. Many people feel that it is unethical to use a control group. However, most studies on cancer screening show that those in the control group are equally likely, if not more likely, to survive in comparison with those who are screened and treated.

Length Bias

Tumors progress at different rates. Some cancers are very slow-growing, while others progress very rapidly. In some cases tumors may regress, remain stable, or progress so slowly that they never produce a clinical problem during an ordinary lifetime. These cases might be described as pseudodisease because they are not clinically significant [19]. The probability that disease is detected through screening is inversely proportional to the rate of progression. For example, with rapidly progressing disease, early detection may not produce a clinical benefit because cases are detected too late. On the other hand, diseases that progress very slowly, with very long preclinical phases, are more likely to be detected by screening. However, it is exactly because they progress so slowly that these detectable diseases may never cause clinical problems.

Figures 5.3 and 5.4 illustrate this issue. The two middle horizontal lines in Fig. 5.3 show the point at which a test can detect a disease (test threshold) and the point at which signs and symptoms of a disease are apparent (clinical threshold). The top horizontal line shows the point at which a patient dies from the disease. The diagonal lines show what happens to four people with rapidly or slowly developing cancers. (The steeper the incline, the more rapid the development of the cancer; Patient "A" has the most rapidly developing disease, and Patient D the slowest.) Patient "A," represented by the leftmost diagonal line, reaches the test and clinical thresholds relatively early, and then goes on to die from the disease. Patient "D," in contrast, represented by the rightmost diagonal, never reaches the test threshold. Before the disease progresses to that point, she dies from another cause. In other words, she never knew she had the disease, but it did not matter because she died of another cause long before the disease would affect her, and even before it would show up on a test. In other words, this patient had what we have earlier described as pseudodisease.

It is useful to consider, in terms of advances in medical technology, how the graph in Fig. 5.3 would be likely to change in the near future. We know that test thresholds are going to go down, as test equipment becomes more sensitive, and as new screening technologies come into widespread use. This inevitable lowering of the test threshold line is shown in Fig. 5.4. Clearly, new tests will be able to detect disease earlier. If we take the same four hypothetical patients with the same type of disease from Fig. 5.3, we see that patient "D" will now most likely be faced with a problem. Even though she is most likely to die of other causes long before she has any signs or symptoms of her disease (at the clinical

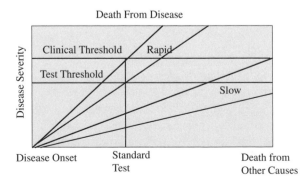

Fig. 5.3 Length Bias. (Adapted from Black and Welch [19])

Fig. 5.4 Length Bias with newer test. With advanced testing the test threshold will be reduced and cases that will never be clinically important will get labeled as disease. (Adapted from Black and Welch [19])

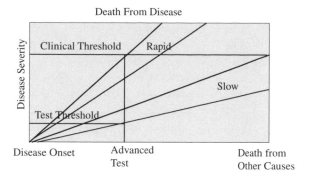

threshold), she will now need to face the fact that she is sick. That knowledge may not do her much good, and it is likely to cause her harm.

Does Screening Find the Wrong Cases?

The rationale for screening is that disease can be caught in its earliest stages. In the case of cancer, this rationale makes at least two important assumptions. First, it assumes that the test will find cancer at early stages. Second, it assumes that early treatment works better than late treatment. Welch challenged both of these basic assumptions [16]. First, he questioned whether screening identifies the most important cases of cancer. Imagine two people with the disease. In one case (Patient B), the disease is very slow-growing and may take 30 or 40 years before it causes death. In the other case (Patient A), the interval between the beginning of the disease and death from cancer is only 6 months. Imagine now that individuals are screened every 5 years. For the slow-growing cancer, the test would identify disease each time it was administered. For a 50-year-old man with prostate cancer, for example, assume the disease was there at the first screening and it was there each time the test was re-administered at ages 55, 60, 65, 70, 75, and 80. Even though the disease was found on each test, it never affected the man's lifestyle, and he died of another cause before he had a chance to die of his cancer.

Patient A had a very rapidly growing cancer that started around age 50 and was detected at age 52, when the disease reached the clinical threshold. The test was unable to identify the disease at age 50, and at the point in time when the man would have been 55 years old, he was no longer alive to be tested. Welch points out that Patient A would have benefited from early detection, while Patient B may have been harmed. (With his slow-growing cancer, Patient B would never have been affected by the disease, but in fact is likely to have received treatment.) In contrast, Patient A may have benefited from treatment, but his cancer would probably not be found early enough by screening, at a point in time when he could be helped.

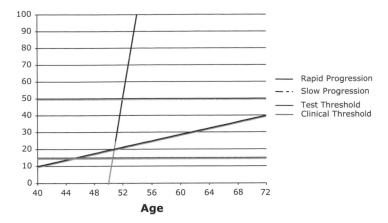

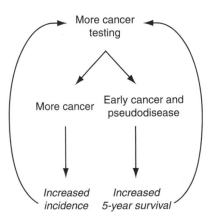

Fig. 5.5 Detection of rapidly progressing and slowing progressing cancers. Slowing progressing cancers may never reach the clinical threshold, but can be detected very early. Rapidly progressing cancers might be missed at screening because they are below the test threshold. However, they progress to severe disease and death rapidly. The most serious cancers are the ones most likely to be overlooked by screening

The perceived benefits of screening often lead to more screening. This is summarized in Fig. 5.6, based on the work of Welch and his colleagues. As shown in the figure, the scheme takes increased cancer testing as a starting point, at the top of the figure. As a result of increased testing, we might find more cancer (indicated on the left side of figure). More cancer detection suggests the development of an "epidemic" of cancer and the need for more aggressive screening. The right side of the figure shows that some of the early cancer detection is actually pseudodisease, which will never result in early death or reduced quality of life. Even though the disease might never have affected a person in his or her lifetime, people with detected cancers now become, after

Fig. 5.6 Screening leads to more screening. (From Welch [16])

testing positive, cancer survivors. Because the disease is detected early, the 5-year-survival rate increases, and this in turn feeds the perception that we are winning the war on cancer. The result: an even more aggressive program to screen for cancer.

What do RCTs on Screening Tell Us?

The best scientific method for the evaluation of cancer screening is to conduct randomized clinical trials (RCTs), in which patients are randomly assigned to screening or to usual care. Table 5.1 summarizes 12 randomized clinical trials, previously reviewed by Black and colleagues [31], in which total mortality was reported. The trials consider a wide variety of screening interventions including screening for breast cancer, screening for colorectal cancer, and screening for lung cancer. Follow-ups ranged from 3 years to over 20 years. The table lists the problem under study, describes the intervention and control conditions, and how many people were studied (noted as n). Finally, it shows the number of disease-specific and all-causes deaths in the intervention condition (noted a I) and the control condition (noted as C). The most striking feature of the table is that, when all causes of death are considered, virtually all of the trials fail to show a benefit of screening. Although the great majority of trials do not support the benefits of screening to reduce total deaths, many authors point to a more positive report on breast screening in New York. This study by Shapiro and colleagues provided the scientific basis for many breast cancer-screening programs. However, among the studies in Table 5.1, the study by Shapiro et al. was the most difficult to interpret because the actual number of people who participated was not clearly reported.

Statisticians and clinical trial experts typically apply the "intention-to-treat" principle. When participants are randomly assigned to treatment or control conditions, they are usually kept in that group for all analyses. This reduces a variety of biases, including biases that result when patients select the treatment they prefer (selection bias). Another problem with the Shapiro study is that it did not use the intention-to-treat principle. About one-third of the treatment group refused to be screened and was eliminated from the analyses. This group had a significantly higher mortality rate and would have further shifted the result away from the benefits of screening.

Table 5.2 summarizes the outcomes of the studies in Table 5.1, excluding the difficult-to-interpret Shapiro study shows the proportion of people who benefited from screening. The table provides information on disease-specific deaths and the so-called all-causes deaths in the intervention and control groups for all interventions. The table also summarizes the all-causes mortality and the proportion of all cases who died in the follow-up interval for the intervention and control groups. Finally, the table summarizes the ARR for disease-specific and for all-causes mortality. The AAR is the proportion of those who died in the

Table 5.1 Summary of clinical trials with reports of total mortality

References	Problem	Intervention	Control	Follow-up	Disease-Specific deaths	All-Causes deaths
Shapiro et al. 1988 [20]	Screening for breast cancer women age 40–64	Mammography plus clinical breast exam n = 30,131(20,128 completed test used in analysis)	Usual care n = 30,565	18 years	I = 263 (1%) C = 307 (1%)	I = 73.7/10,000 person years C = 75.4/10,000 person years
Laszlotabar et al. 1989	Screening for breast cancer	Mammography n = 77,080	Not invited for screening n = 55,985	7.9 years	I = 160 C = 167	I = 6,899 C = 5,085
Andersson et al. 1998 [21]	Screening for breast cancer in women aged >45	Five rounds of Mammography at intervals of 18–24 months n = 21,088	Not invited for screening n = 21,195	8.8 years	I = 63 C = 66	I = 1,777 C = 1,809
Bjurstam et al. 1997 [22]	Screening for breast cancer in women aged <50	2-view mammography 18-month interval n = 11,724	Not screened until 6–7 year n = 14,217	10 years	I = 18 C = 40	I = 409 C = 506
Roberts et al. 1990 [23]	Screening for breast cancer in women aged 45–64	Oblique and carniocaudal view mammography; Clinical examination n = 23,226	Not invited for screening n = 21,904	7 years	I = 68 C = 76	I = 1274 C = 1,490
Miller et al. 1992 [24] 2002	Screening for breast cancer in women aged 40–49	Mammography; Physical examination of the breasts n = 25,214	Single physical examination of the breasts n = 25,216	11–16 years	(To end of 1996) I = 105 (C = 108	(To end of 1993) I = 413 C = 413
Miller et al. 2000 [25]	Screening for breast cancer in women aged 50–59	Annual 2-view mammography (craniocaudal & mediolateral oblique views); Annual physical exam; Taught self-exam n = 19,711	Physical exam only n = 19,694	13 years	I = 88 (11.9%); C = 90 (12.9%)	I = 647 (88.1%); C = 600 (87.1%)

Table 5.1 (continued)

References	Problem	Intervention	Control	Follow-up	Disease-Specific deaths	All-Causes deaths
Mandel et al. 2000 [26]	Screening for colorectal cancer in people aged 50–80	Fecal occult blood test with rehydration; Tested Annually: I_1 = 15,570 Tested Biennally: I_2 = 15,587	Not invited for screening n = 15,394	13 years	I_1 = 121 I_2 = 148 C = 177	I_1 = 5,236 I_2 = 5,213 C = 5,186
Harcastle et al. 1996 [27]	Screening for colorectal cancer in people aged 45–76	Fecal occult blood screening n = 76,466	Not invited for screening n = 76,384	7.8 years	I = 360 C = 420	I = 12,624 C = 12,515
Kronborg et al. 1996 [28]	Screening for colorectoral cancer in people aged 45–75	Fecal occult blood screening (Biennial Hemocult II without rehydration) n = 30,967	Not invited for screening n = 30,966	10 years	I = 205 C = 249	I = 6,228 C = 6,303
Kubik et al. [29] 1990	Screening for lung cancer in cigarette-smoking males aged 40–64	6-monthly screening by chest x-ray and sputum cytology n = 3,171	No asymptomatic investigation n = 3174	5 years including 3 years of annual chest x-rays	I = 85 C = 67	I = 341 C = 293
Marcus et al. 2000 [30]	Screening for lung cancer	Chest x-ray; Sputum cytology n = 4,618	Usual care n = 4,593	20.5 years	I = 337 C = 303	I = 2,493 C = 2,445

Table 5.2 Disease-specific and All-causes mortality and AARs for RCTs of screening

Reference	Proportion dead from specific cause intervention	Proportion dead from specific cause control	ARR specific	Proportion dead from all-causes intervention	Proportion dean from all-causes control	ARR all causes
Laszlotabar et al. 1989	0.002	0.003	0.001	0.092	0.094	0.002
Andersson et al. 1998 [21]	0.003	0.003	0.000	0.087	0.088	0.001
Bjurstam et al. 1997 [22]	0.002	0.003	0.001	0.036	0.037	0.000
Roberts et al. 1990 [23]	0.003	0.003	0.001	0.058	0.071	0.013
Miller et al. 1992 [24]	0.004	0.004	0.000	0.021	0.021	0.000
Miller et al. 2000 [25]	0.004	0.005	0.000	0.037	0.035	−0.002
Mandel et al. 2000 [26]	0.008	0.011	0.004	0.344	0.345	0.001
Harcastle et al. 1996 [27]	0.005	0.005	0.001	0.170	0.169	−0.001
Kronborg et al. 1996 [28]	0.007	0.008	0.001	0.208	0.210	0.002
Kubik et al. [29] 1990	0.027	0.021	−0.006	0.134	0.119	−0.015
Marcus et al. 2000 [30]	0.073	0.066	−0.007	0.613	0.606	−0.007

control group minus the proportion who died in the intervention group (see Chapter 3). If the number is positive, there is a benefit of screening; when the number is negative, screening may cause harm. As the table shows, the ARR for all-causes mortality is remarkably small. Among 11 trials, 5 had overall mortality in the direction opposite direction to what was expected and 6 had overall mortality in the expected direction. However, in nearly all trials the ARR was near 0. When screening helps people, it is often only one or two people per hundred thousand screened who get the benefit. In other words, there is little evidence from these trials to suggest that screening leads to longer life.

Two features shown in Tables 5.1 and 5.2 are especially important. If cancer-screening tests really provide benefit, then we would expect those who were screened to have a longer life expectancy than those who were not. As the tables show, it is quite remarkable that cancer-screening trials have been unable to document that people who are screened live any longer than those who are not screened [31]. We call this the "total mortality issue" because it focuses on total life expectancy. Advocates for cancer screening recognize that there is no total mortality benefit but argue that there are benefits for deaths from specific types of cancer [32]. The center columns in Table 5.2 show the outcomes for specific types of cancer for screened and unscreened patients. For colorectal cancer, for example, there is a disease-specific benefit. This means that those screened are significantly less likely to die of colorectal cancer than those who are not screened.

The argument against considering all-causes mortality is that the benefits of screening appear diluted. The apparent impact of any benefit for what, in the big picture, is essentially a rare cause of death will seem very small when it is presented in a set of data containing a large amount of "noise." The Minnesota colon-cancer-screening trial offers perhaps the best example [26]. Patients were randomly assigned to occult blood screening annually ($n = 15,570$), biennially ($n = 15,587$), or to usual care ($n = 15,394$). Over the 18-year period, the death rate from colon or rectal cancer (CRC) was approximately 10 per 1,000, or 1 percent. Over the same time period, the all-causes death rate was approximately 340 per 1,000, or 34 percent. Suppose a reasonable expectation for screening is that it will reduce CRC deaths by 30 percent—that is, from 1.0 percent to 0.7 percent, or 7 per 1,000 from 10 per 1,000. Suppose, furthermore, that screening is expected to have no effect on deaths from causes other than CRC—that is, that screening is expected to reduce the overall death rate from 34 percent to 33.7 percent.

If the study was designed to have an 80 percent chance of observing a statistically significant decline in CRC deaths, and if the true change is 0.3 percent, we would need approximately 15,000 participants in each of two arms, or a total of 30,000 people. To get the same power in measuring a 0.3 percent decline in the *total* death rate, we would need a study that included approximately 385,000 in each arm, or 770,000 participants.

Some would argue that a 0.3-percent decrease in death is too small to be concerned about. Others would say that 0.3-percent decline in the all-causes death rate is a significant health benefit, but only if we can demonstrate conclusively that this decline actually occurs. If we can get enough money to do a controlled study of screening that includes 770,000 people, we can be reasonably confident of determining whether screening has an effect on all-causes mortality. If it is demonstrated to have an effect, and if the screening is determined to be "cost-effective," then we should be comfortable in recommending widespread screening programs. However, doing the study would cost hundreds of millions of dollars.

Even though CRL affects only a small number of people, there are many diseases that result in death for a relatively small portion of the population. It does not make sense to say that because these diseases kill a relatively small number of people ("only" 1 percent of the population), that we should not care about figuring out how to prevent or treat them.

But we, must face the nagging public-health question. With small benefits and some potential for harm, what are we comfortable recommending? We will explore that issue in the following sections.

Evidence-Based Medicine Approach

To push this debate one step further, imagine what if you are using the results of the Minnesota study to determine whether or not we should be screening for colon or rectal cancer. Figure 5.7 shows the number of deaths from colon and rectal cancer per thousand participants in the study. The results look quite impressive. However, Fig. 5.8 shows the deaths from all causes in the Minnesota

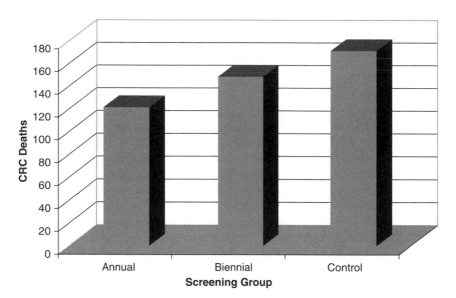

Fig. 5.7 Number of colon or rectal cancer deaths 18 years after random assignment to usual care or to occult blood screening either annually or biennially in the Minnesota colon-cancer-screening trail

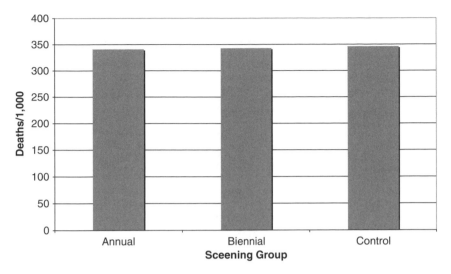

Fig. 5.8 Number of deaths from all causes 18 years after random assignment to usual care or to occult blood screening either annually or biennially in the Minnesota colon-cancer-screening trail

study. In contrast to Fig. 5.7, Fig. 5.8 suggests that there is no advantage of screening for extending your life expectancy. The chances of dying of colon and rectal cancer are reduced by less than one percent and the chances of living longer are not changed at all. Even under the best of circumstances, the number of people that we would need to screen to have one positive outcome is about 268. This screening example is interesting because it shows how different interpretations can come from the very same data. The Minnesota study has been taken as the best evidence that we need to have national screening programs for colon and rectal cancer. On the other hand, the same evidence can be used to suggest that colon and rectal cancer screening has essentially no public health benefit.

Interpretation of Cancer-Screening Evidence by Peer Panels

Professional groups that have reviewed the clinical evidence often disagree about the value of screening. For example, there are no studies that show a clear benefit from receiving a PSA test because completing the test does not appear to result in a reduction in overall mortality. However, treatment for prostate cancer (typically surgical removal of the tumor) carries with it a significant risk of impotence and incontinence [33]. Hence, receiving a PSA test may result in a reduction in quality of life [34]. Recognizing these uncertainties, most professional groups now recommend some sort of shared decision

Table 5.3 Summary of recommendations for PSA screening

Group	Recommendation	Reference
US Preventive Services Taskforce (USPSTF)	Do not screen	35
American College of Physicians-American Society of Internal Medicine (ACP-ASIM)	Share decision-making with patient	36
American Academy of Family Physicians (AAFP)	Share decision-making with patient	37
American Urological Association (AUA)	Offer screening if life expectancy > 10 years	38
American Cancer Society	Screen except for men with short life expectancy	39

making for PSA screening. Table 5.3 summarizes the recommendations from several groups. All of these are serious and reputable organizations—but the organizations have wide divergences in their recommendations.

Another example of differences of opinion between professional groups concerns the age for initiating screening for breast cancer using mammography [40–43]. Among women between the ages of 50 and 74, periodic screening results in significantly lower rates of death from breast cancer [44]. However, there is very little evidence that screening is of benefit to women younger than age 50. Nonetheless, in February 2002, the US Department of Health and Human Services endorsed mammography for women 40 years of age and older as evidence of commitment to preventive medicine. It is widely believed, however, that the public-health benefit of promoting screening mammography for women between 40 and 50 years of age may be somewhat limited. All clinical trials and meta-analyses have failed to show a population benefit of screening women in this age group [40–43, 45, 46].

Earlier, in January 1997, the US National Institutes of Health (NIH) had convened a panel to make recommendations about the use of screening mammography for women 40–50 years of age. Noting that no convincing evidence showed benefits of screening younger women, the committee recommended against pre-menopausal screening. Yet, the conclusions of the panel were rebuffed by the American Cancer Society. Richard Klausner, then the director of the National Cancer Institute of the National Institutes of Health, decided to disregard the report of his own expert panel. Shortly thereafter, the American Cancer Society appointed a panel of experts chosen because each expert already believed that screening was valuable for 40- to 50-year-old women, and not surprisingly, this new panel recommended that the target population for screening should be enlarged [46].

The controversy died down for a brief time but reemerged in 2001, when Olsen and Gotzsche reanalyzed earlier trials and classified studies by methodological quality [47]. Their analysis noted that the only studies supporting screening mammography for women of any age were of low quality and that those studies not supporting screening mammography tended to have greater

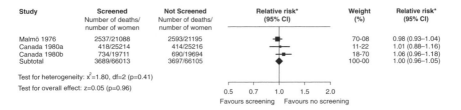

Study	Screened	Not Screened	Relative risk*	Weight	Relative risk*
	Number of deaths/ number of women	Number of deaths/ number of women	(95% CI)	(%)	(95% CI)
Malmö 1976	2537/21088	2593/21195		70-08	0.98 (0.93–1.04)
Canada 1980a	418/25214	414/25216		11-22	1.01 (0.88–1.16)
Canada 1980b	734/19711	690/19694		18-70	1.06 (0.96–1.18)
Subtotal	3689/66013	3697/66105		100-00	1.00 (0.96–1.05)

Test for heterogeneity: x^2=1.80, df=2 (p=0.41)

Test for overall effect: z=0.05 (p=0.96)

0.5   0.7   1.0   1.5   2.0
Favours screening   Favours no screening

Fig. 5.9 Relative risk and confidence intervals for mammography RCTs. A relative risk less than 1.0 favors screening, while a relative risk greater than 1.0 favors no screening. The size of the symbols reflects the relative number of people in the study. Confidence intervals are used to estimate whether the relative risk ratio is statistically significant. To be significant, the interval cannot include 1.0. In this set of studies none of the studies was statistically significant because the interval included 1.0 in all cases. (From Olsen and Gotzsche [47].)

methodological rigor. The findings are summarized in Fig. 5.9. Remarkably, there appeared to be no benefit at all for screening—the relative risk ratio was nearly 1.0.

Even though many scholars agree with Olsen and Gotzsche, the controversy about the usefulness of early mammography continues. Considering the seriousness of the disease, and the widespread fear it creates, the controversy should come as no surprise. In an effort to shed some light, we take a closer look at some of the numbers in the next section of this chapter.

The Mammography Paradox

A variety of studies have shown that more breast cancer is diagnosed in screened than in unscreened women [48]. It is assumed that undetected cancer will progress and eventually cause early death. Despite the popularity of this belief, it is not well supported by data. Averaged across the seven major clinical trials that provided enough information for reanalysis, there appears very little benefit of screening. This is best summarized in a graphic from Baines [49] (Fig. 5.10). The figure suggests that screened women (solid line) are actually more likely to die for the first 11 years following mammography than women in the control group (broken line). After that, there appears to be a reduction in mortality for screened women, but the effects overall are not statistically significant.

How could it be possible that women who are screened are no better off, or even worse off than women who are not screened? One possibility is that some tumors get better on their own. Several investigators have suggested that some tumors spontaneously regress [50]. Because breast cancer is rarely left untreated, we know surprisingly little about the natural history of the disease. In one analysis, Vahl, Maehlan, and Welch [51] attempted to piece together the natural history of breast cancer. They used a creative method for comparing

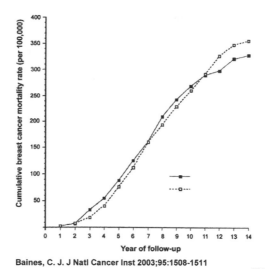

Baines, C. J. J Natl Cancer Inst 2003;95:1508-1511

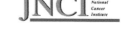

Fig. 5.10 Overall cumulative breast cancer mortality rates per 100,000 women aged 40–49 in intervention and control groups from several trials of breast cancer screening. (From Baines [49])

age-matched groups of women living in four Norwegian counties. In 1996, these areas of Norway began screening women with mammography every other year. In the analysis, they considered the group that was screened three different times between 1996 and 2001. Eligibility was defined as being between the ages of 50 and 64 in 1996. For a comparison, they used women who were between the ages of 50 and 64 in 1992. In other words, rather than going to another locale to compare results, they went to another segment of time to get their comparison group. These women would have been screened three times between 1992 and 1997 if there had been a program. The women in the comparison group were all invited to receive a one-time prevalence mammogram. The "prevalence" mammogram is used to get a snapshot of how many women have breast cancer at any particular point in time. In this case, a sample of women were invited for a test once the larger screening program began. In summary, the screened group had three mammograms while the comparison group had only one mammogram. Because of the slight time overlap of the two groups, the mammogram for the control group was given at the same age as the third mammogram for the screened group. We would expect, then, that the prevalence of breast cancer should be the same in the two groups. However, that is not what happened. The analysis suggested that incidences of invasive breast cancer were 22 percent higher in the screened group than in the comparison group. This result is summarized in Fig. 5.11.

How might we explain this result? Panel B shows that the odds ratio for invasive cancer within 6 years is 22 percent higher in the screened group in

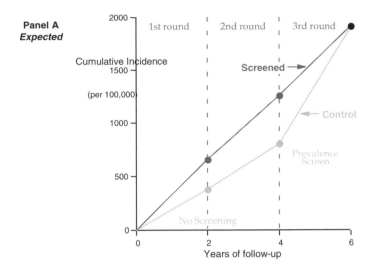

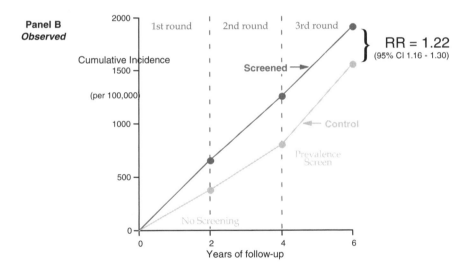

Fig. 5.11 Expected and observed cumulative incidence of invasive breast cancer among women who receive biennial screening versus controls who receive only a prevalence screening at the end of their observation period. *Panel A* shows what would be expected given the conventional model of cancer progression: invasive breast cancers in the control group that would have been detected by regular screening ultimately either progress to be detected clinically or persist to be detected by the prevalence screen. Thus, the 6-year cumulative incidence would be the same in both groups. *Panel B* shows what was observed in our study: a deficit in cumulative incidence persists in the control group following the prevalence screen. (From Zahl et al. [51])

comparison with the group that was not screened, since it summarizes or crystallizes the oddity of the result. The authors believe that some breast cancers must spontaneously regress or even disappear. We would expect that screened and unscreened women would have the same number of tumors eventually detected. However, it appears that those screened on a regular basis have more tumors. Not only do these women have these cancers detected, but they also get treatment. This study suggests that had these cancers not been treated, some would have gone away on their own or at least diminished to a size at which they would become undetectable.

The observation that screened women can have poorer outcomes than nonscreened women has been described as the mammography paradox. The paradox has received relatively little attention because, on the surface, it makes little sense. How could it be that women who have cancer diagnosed early are more likely to die of breast cancer than those who have their disease detected later? One explanation comes from a group of vascular biologists and surgeons [52]. They suggest that surgery might actually increase the chances of breast cancer recurrence because it induces angiogenesis, or the development of increased blood flow. In order to evaluate this hypothesis, they studied the likelihood of relapse following surgery for breast cancer in women between the ages of 40 and 49. They discovered that relapses are common between 8 and 10 months following surgery for younger women with node-positive breast cancer. Using a computer model, they concluded that many women have small micro-tumors in areas of the breast close to the tumor that was extracted through surgery. These micro-tumors might have regressed on their own if undisturbed. However, the invasive surgery may have stimulated increased blood flow that ultimately nourished the micro-tumors. The computer simulation suggested that this model could explain the mammography paradox for women 40–49 years of age.

In summary, evaluating the benefits of screening is quite challenging. Some evidence suggests that women who are screened for breast cancer may actually be more likely to die of breast cancer than those not screened, but a word of caution is in order. The increase in mortality has not been shown in all studies, and the increase in deaths that has been observed is very small. Nevertheless, there is a reason for some concern. It is possible that aggressive screening and treatment may cause some problems. It will take time and more studies to figure this out. I understand that women want answers now, but the picture is unfortunately more complicated that it appears to be on first glance.

How Many Screening Tests are Needed to Prevent a Death?

In medical and public-health statistics, the NNT is the number of people you would need to be treated or tested in order to prevent 1 bad outcome. In Chapter 3 we introduced this concept along with the concept of ARR. The

NNT is 1.0 divided by the ARR. Using data from the United States Preventive Services Task Force, Gates estimated the number of people one would need to screen for various cancers in order to prevent one death. The task force had previously evaluated the quality of statistical evidence using letter grades. The strongest evidence, which offers the most confidence in the recommendation, is given an "A," while the evidence leaving the greatest level of uncertainty is given a "D." Quality of evidence is judged by the committees' view of the design of the study. Good-quality evidence is noted as Level I, while limited quality evidence is noted as Level II. Level III is reserved for other nonsystematic evidence. The summary is shown in Table 5.4. The task force concluded that there is not enough evidence to support screening for prostate cancer using the PSA test or to screen for lung cancer using the chest X-ray. The best evidence supported the use of pap smears and mammography for women older than 50. However, even using the most optimistic evidence, screening mammography for women from ages 40 through 49 looked questionable. According to the analysis, we would need to screen 3,125 women every other year to prevent one bad outcome. And, this analysis uses the most optimistic data on the benefits of screening. Several analysts who have reviewed the evidence on mammography for younger women see no benefit at all. In other words, the number of women we would need to be screened is infinite.

Variations in Screening Rates and Impacts on Healthcare Costs

The number of cancer-screening tests offered is considered an indicator of quality healthcare. In fact, health plans are often evaluated by the proportion of patients who receive cancer-screening tests. We also know that rates of screening differ by community. For instance, cancer-screening rates are increasing, and the number of cases identified early has gone up [54]. Communities with lower average income and education tend to get less screening than communities where most of the people are affluent. This has lead to calls to spend more money providing cancer screening for the medically underserved [54]. However, do we know that there is a health disadvantage for those living in communities where screening is less common?

There is substantial geographic variability in the rate of cancer screening. For example, analysis of Medicare claims by Wennberg and colleagues [55] shows that in Michigan and Florida, mammograms are done routinely. In Lansing, Michigan, nearly 35 percent of all women older than age 65 had received mammograms, and similarly high rates were observed in Fort Lauderdale and Sarasota, Florida. On the other hand, only 13 percent of the women in Oklahoma City had obtained mammograms and a variety of cities had similar rates. Salt Lake, for example, had a rate of 13.4 percent [55]. If screening provides benefit, outcomes should be better in areas that use more screening. In areas where screening is done more often, more cases of breast cancer are

Table 5.4 Summary of Cancer-Screening tests. (From Gates [53])

Test	Strength of recommendation*	Quality of evidence*	RRR†	NNS‡	Controversies
Pap smear for cervical cancer	A	II-2, II-3	>0.80	1,140	Interval, new technologies, when to stop
Mammography					
Age>50 years	A	I, II-2	0.23	543	Interval (annual vs. biannual), when to stop
Age 40–49 years	C	I	0.08	3,125	Some evidence of significant reduction with follow-up > 10 years; false-positives
FOBT for colorectal cancer	B	I	0.15–0.20	588–1,000	Interval (annual vs. biannual), compliance, role of sigmoidoscopy, cost/benefit
PSA for prostate cancer	D	II-2	NA	NA	Unproven; RCTs in progress
Chest film for lung cancer	D	I, II-1	NA	NA	Recent reports of spiral CT for screening may reopen controversy

Pap = Papanicolaou; FOBT = fecal occult blood test; PSA = prostate-specific antigen; RCTs = randomized clinical trials; NA = not applicable; CT = computed tomography.

* Per U.S. Preventive Services Task Force rating (see Table 5.3).

† RRR = relative risk reduction: the proportion of deaths from the cancer in question in the control group that could have been prevented by the screening intervention.

‡ NNS = number of patients needed to screen over a 10-year period to prevent one death from the cancer in question. Calculated as the reciprocal of the absolute risk reduction.

found. However, there appears to be no relationship between these screening rates and mortality rates from breast cancer [55]. Similarly, PSA screening is done much more commonly in the Pacific Northwest region of the US than it is in New England communities, such as New Haven, CT. Although many more cases are found and treated in the Pacific Northwest, there is no evidence of reduced mortality due to prostate cancer in these regions [55]. More screening finds more cases but appears unrelated to better health outcomes.

Conclusions

Cancer screening remains a highly controversial topic. For nearly a century, charitable organizations have promoted early detection as the key to cancer prevention. However, evidence does not always support the value of early detection.

Yet, a disease-reservoir hypothesis would argue that although the disease is very common, particularly among older adults, much of it is pseudodisease: That is, much of this disease will never be clinically relevant because it will not affect life expectancy or reduce quality of life. Many cases of cancer detected through screening might be pseudodisease because the affected patients would have never known about the problem during their lifetimes.

Two important problems keep the controversy about cancer screening alive. One is that randomized clinical trials fail to show the benefits of screening in terms of total mortality. Even trials that show disease-specific mortality benefits often do not show that screening extends life expectancy. A second problem is that the development of better biomarkers and improvements in screening methodology may make the problem more severe. Improved screening methodologies may identify more pseudodisease, and few new technologies clearly distinguish between it and true, clinically significant disease. It is unknown whether many current biomarkers are related to diseases that shorten life expectancy or reduce quality of life. Systematic research is necessary to document the validity of these new outcome measures. There appears to be a disconnect between the advocacy for screening by the American Cancer Society and the scientific evidence supporting screening.

And a final concern is that screening is expensive. If we devote healthcare resources to screening programs, fewer resources are available for other prevention programs. Prevention works, but many preventive programs are underfunded or unfunded. Many administrators use screening as the poster child of their prevention portfolio. Perhaps it is time to move some of the prevention budget to other proven activities, such as tobacco control or exercise programs.

References

1. Schwartz LM, Woloshin S, Fowler FJ, Jr., Welch HG. Enthusiasm for cancer screening in the United States. *JAMA*. Jan 7 2004;291(1):71–78.
2. Aronowitz RA. Do not delay: breast cancer and time, 1900–1970. *Milbank Q*. 2001; 79(3):355–386, III.
3. Eddy DM. The frequency of cervical cancer screening. Comparison of a mathematical model with empirical data. *Cancer*. Sep 1 1987;60(5):1117–1122.
4. Harris P, Carnes M. Is there an age at which we should stop performing screening pap smears and mammography? *Cleve Clin J Med*. Apr 2002;69(4):272–273.
5. Parnes BL, Smith PC, Conry CM, Domke H. When should we stop mammography screening for breast cancer in elderly women? *J Fam Pract*. Feb 2001;50(2):110–111.
6. Shapiro S, Coleman EA, Broeders M, et al. Breast cancer screening programmes in 22 countries: current policies, administration and guidelines. International Breast Cancer Screening Network (IBSN) and the European Network of Pilot Projects for Breast Cancer Screening. *Int J Epidemiol*. Oct 1998;27(5):735–742.
7. Kaplan RM. Shared medical decision making. A new tool for preventive medicine. *Am J Prev Med*. Jan 2004;26(1):81–83.
8. Arnold K. Mammography guidelines in the national spotlight again. *J Natl Cancer Inst*. Mar 20 2002;94(6):411–413.
9. Screening for prostate cancer: commentary on the recommendations of the Canadian Task Force on the Periodic Health Examination. The U.S. Preventive Services Task Force. *Am J Prev Med*. Jul–Aug 1994;10(4):187–193.
10. Levenson D. Routine prostate screening may be unnecessary and harmful. *Rep Med Guidel Outcomes Res*. Jan 10 2003;14(1):5–7.
11. Weston R, Parr N. New NHS guidelines for PSA testing in primary care. *Lancet*. Jan 4 2003;361(9351):89–90.
12. Farhat WA, Habbal AA, Khauli RB. A guideline to clinical utility of prostate specific antigen. *Saudi Med J*. Mar 2000;21(3):223–227.
13. New PSA guidelines for older men. *Johns Hopkins Med Lett Health After 50*. Sep 1998;10(7):1–2.
14. Duperray B, Junrod B. Depistage du cancer du sein. *Medecine*. 2006;2:364–367.
15. American Cancer Society. California Division, California Cancer Registry. California cancer facts & figures. Oakland, CA: American Cancer Society California Division 2008.
16. Welch HG. *Should I Be Tested for Cancer?* Berkeley, CA: University of California Press; 2004.
17. Black WC, Welch HG. Screening for disease. *AJR Am J Roentgenol*. Jan 1997;168(1): 3–11.
18. Welch HG, Black WC. Evaluating randomized trials of screening. *J Gen Intern Med*. Feb 1997;12(2):118–124.
19. Black WC, Welch HG. Advances in diagnostic imaging and overestimations of disease prevalence and the benefits of therapy. *N Engl J Med*. Apr 29 1993;328(17):1237–1243.
20. Tabar L, Fagerberg G, Duffy SW, Day NE. The Swedish two county trial of mammographic screening for breast cancer: recent results and calculation of benefit. *J Epidemiol Community Health*. Jun 1989;43(2):107–114.
21. Andersson I, Aspegren K, Janzon L, et al. Mammographic screening and mortality from breast cancer: the Malmo mammographic screening trial. *BMJ*. Oct 15 1988;297(6654): 943–948.
22. Bjurstam N, Bjorneld L, Duffy SW, et al. The Gothenburg breast screening trial: first results on mortality, incidence, and mode of detection for women ages 39–49 years at randomization. *Cancer*. Dec 1 1997;80(11):2091–2099.
23. Roberts MM, Alexander FE, Anderson TJ, et al. Edinburgh trial of screening for breast cancer: mortality at seven years. *Lancet*. Feb 3 1990;335(8684):241–246.

24. Miller AB, Baines CJ, To T, Wall C. Canadian National Breast Screening Study: 1. Breast cancer detection and death rates among women aged 40–49 years. *Cmaj.* Nov 15 1992;147(10):1459–1476.

25. Miller AB, To T, Baines CJ, Wall C. Canadian National Breast Screening Study-2: 13-year results of a randomized trial in women aged 50–59 years. *J Natl Cancer Inst.* Sep 20 2000;92(18):1490–1499.

26. Mandel JS, Church TR, Ederer F, Bond JH. Colorectal cancer mortality: effectiveness of biennial screening for fecal occult blood. *J Natl Cancer Inst.* Mar 3 1999;91(5):434–437.

27. Hardcastle JD, Chamberlain JO, Robinson MH, et al. Randomised controlled trial of faecal-occult-blood screening for colorectal cancer. *Lancet.* Nov 30 1996;348(9040): 1472–1477.

28. Kronborg O, Fenger C, Olsen J, Jorgensen OD, Sondergaard O. Randomised study of screening for colorectal cancer with faecal-occult-blood test. *Lancet.* Nov 30 1996; 348(9040):1467–1471.

29. Kubik A, Parkin DM, Khlat M, Erban J, Polak J, Adamec M. Lack of benefit from semi-annual screening for cancer of the lung: follow-up report of a randomized controlled trial on a population of high-risk males in Czechoslovakia. *Int J Cancer.* Jan 15 1990;45(1): 26–33.

30. Marcus PM, Bergstralh EJ, Fagerstrom RM, et al. Lung cancer mortality in the Mayo Lung Project: impact of extended follow-up. *J Natl Cancer Inst.* Aug 16 2000;92(16): 1308–1316.

31. Black WC, Haggstrom DA, Welch HG. All-cause mortality in randomized trials of cancer screening. *J Natl Cancer Inst.* Feb 6 2002;94(3):167–173.

32. de Koning HJ. Mammographic screening: evidence from randomised controlled trials. *Ann Oncol.* Aug 2003;14(8):1185–1189.

33. Barry MJ. Early detection and aggressive treatment of prostate cancer: groping in the dark. [Comment On: J Gen Intern Med. 2000 Oct;15(10):739–48]. *J Gen Int Med.* 2000;15(10):749–751.

34. Barry MJ. PSA screening for prostate cancer: the current controversy–a viewpoint. Patient Outcomes Research Team for Prostatic Diseases [see comments]. *Ann Oncol.* 1998;9(12):1279–1282.

35. U.S. Preventive Services Task Force, United States. Office of Disease Prevention and Health Promotion. *Guide to clinical preventive services: report of the U.S. Preventive Services Task Force.* 2nd ed. Washington, DC: U.S. Dept. of Health and Human Services Office of Public Health and Science Office of Disease Prevention and Health Promotion: Supt. of Docs. U.S. G.P.O. distributor; 1996.

36. Screening for prostate cancer. American College of Physicians [see comments]. *Ann Intern Med.* 1997;126(6):480–484.

37. Physicians. AAoF. Summary of policy reddommendations for periodic health examinations. www.aafp.org.exam/pos_gen_guide.html. 2000.

38. Prostate-specific antigen (PSA) best practice policy. American Urological Association (AUA). *Oncology.* 2000;14(2):267–272, 277–268, 280 passim.

39. Society AC. *Prostate Cancer: Treatment Guidelines for Patients Version II.* Atlanta: American Cancer Society; 2001.

40. McLellan F. Independent US panel fans debate on mammography. *Lancet.* Feb 2 2002;359(9304):409.

41. Miettinen OS, Henschke CI, Pasmantier MW, Smith JP, Libby DM, Yankelevitz DF. Mammographic screening: no reliable supporting evidence? *Lancet.* Feb 2 2002; 359(9304):404–405.

42. Nystrom L, Andersson I, Bjurstam N, Frisell J, Nordenskjold B, Rutqvist LE. Long-term effects of mammography screening: updated overview of the Swedish randomised trials. *Lancet.* Mar 16 2002;359(9310):909–919.

43. Gelmon KA, Olivotto I. The mammography screening debate: time to move on. *Lancet.* Mar 16 2002;359(9310):904–905.
44. Navarro AM, Kaplan RM. Mammography screening: prospects and opportunity costs. *Womens Health.* Winter 1996;2(4):209–233.
45. Barton MB, Moore S, Polk S, Shtatland E, Elmore JG, Fletcher SW. Increased patient concern after false-positive mammograms: clinician documentation and subsequent ambulatory visits. *J Gen Intern Med.* Mar 2001;16(3):150–156.
46. Fletcher SW. Whither scientific deliberation in health policy recommendations? Alice in the Wonderland of breast-cancer screening. *N Engl J Med.* Apr 17 1997;336(16): 1180–1183.
47. Olsen O, Gotzsche PC. Cochrane review on screening for breast cancer with mammography. *Lancet.* Oct 20 2001;358(9290):1340–1342.
48. Barratt A, Howard K, Irwig L, Salkeld G, Houssami N. Model of outcomes of screening mammography: information to support informed choices. *BMJ.* Apr 23 2005;330 (7497):936.
49. Baines CJ. Mammography screening: are women really giving informed consent? *J Natl Cancer Inst.* Oct 15 2003;95(20):1508–1511.
50. Zahl PH, Maehlen J. Model of outcomes of screening mammography: spontaneous regression of breast cancer may not be uncommon. *BMJ.* Aug 6 2005;331(7512):350; author reply 351.
51. Zahl P, Mæhlen J, Welch H. The Natural History of Invasive Breast Cancers Detected by Screening Mammography. *Arch Intern Med.* Nov 24 2008.
52. Baum M, Demicheli R, Hrushesky W, Retsky M. Does surgery unfavourably perturb the "natural history" of early breast cancer by accelerating the appearance of distant metastases? *Eur J Cancer.* Mar 2005;41(4):508–515.
53. Gates TJ. Screening for cancer: evaluating the evidence. *Am. Family Physician,* 2001; 63(3):513–522.
54. Andersen LD, Remington PL, Trentham-Dietz A, Robert S. Community trends in the early detection of breast cancer in Wisconsin, 1980–1998. *Am J Prev Med.* Jan 2004;26(1): 51–55.
55. Wennberg JE. *The Dartmouth Atlas of Health Care in the United States.* Hanover, NH: Trustees of Dartmouth College; 1998.

Chapter 6
Deciding When Blood Pressure Is Too High

In 1992 Geoffrey Rose published *The Strategy of Preventive Medicine* [1]. Many consider the book to be one of the most important statements about epidemiology and public health written in the twentieth century. Rose was particularly concerned about disease of the coronary arteries that supply blood to the heart. Doctors describe occlusion of these large arteries as coronary heart disease (CHD) or just coronary disease. Heart attacks typically result from disease within these coronary arteries.

Rose noted that there are systematic relationships between risk factors for heart disease and poor health outcomes. High blood presume is one of the most important risk factors. For example, the relationship between systolic blood pressure (SBP) and both heart attack and stroke become systematically more likely beginning with SBPs above 110 mmHg [2, 3]. More recently, a major study on cholesterol-lowering, known as the Heart Protection Study, demonstrated that lowering LDL cholesterol using simvastatin (Zocor) reduced the development of vascular disease independent of the initial levels of serum cholesterol [4].

We usually assume that most heart attacks and strokes are suffered by people with the highest levels of blood pressure. Rose argued that only small portions of heart attacks or strokes occur in those with risk factor scores above typical therapeutic thresholds—the point at which medical treatment is initiated. In the days when Rose was trained as a physician, the point at which therapy for high blood pressure was initiated for SBP was as high as 160 mmHg. The point of treatment initiation is called the therapeutic threshold. For example, in contrast to those with a SBP less than 120 mmHg, only about 24 percent of the deaths from stroke accrue to those with SBPs higher than 160 mmHg [5], which was the standard therapeutic threshold. The great majority of heart attacks and strokes occur for those with risk factor scores below the usual thresholds for the initiation of treatment.

In clinical medicine, the usual protocol requires the measurement of blood pressure during an office visit and application of medicine to those with clinically defined hypertension. Too much attention, according to Rose, has been devoted to case identification and treatment, and not enough attention has been paid to shifting the therapeutic threshold curves for blood pressure and cholesterol

R.M. Kaplan, *Disease, Diagnoses, and Dollars*, DOI 10.1007/978-0-387-74045-4_6,
© Springer Science+Business Media, LLC 2009

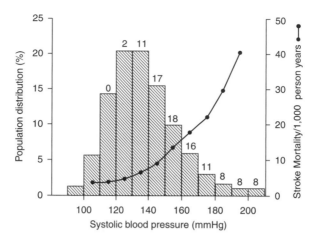

Fig. 6.1 Population systolic pressure and stroke in the Whitehall Study. The bars on the graph are the age-adjusted numbers of people in the population at each level of blood pressure. The scale for this variable is shown on the left side of the graph. The line on the graph is for stroke death rates for each 1,000 persons in the population. The scale for deaths is shown on the right side of the graph. (This figure was originally published in Marmot and Poulter [5]. Copyright Elsevier, 2002.)

downward [6]. In fact, Rose went a step further. He argued that, instead of treating some people, we should treat all people—the entire population.

This argument is summarized in Fig. 6.1. The line in the figure shows the relationship between SBP and stroke mortality. As blood pressure gets higher, the chances that an individual will have a stroke increase. The bars on the graph show the actual number of strokes in the population. Very few people have extremely high blood pressure. Rose argued that most people benefit from having their blood pressure lowered. Since more people have average levels of blood pressure, a larger number of lives will be saved by attending to everyone, rather than the clinical approach of attending only to the most extreme cases. A population-based intervention that shifts the distribution of blood-pressure treatment toward the left—that is, to include those with lower SBP—will have greater impact on population health than will targeted screening [5]. This argument forms the basis for contemporary thinking about population-based preventive medicine.

Rose argued that population-based preventive measures must meet several criteria. First, they must be low-cost. Second, they must be minimally invasive. Any intervention applied to an entire population must produce as little pain and discomfort as possible. The diagnostic threshold is the point along a continuum above which values are believed to represent disease. The diagnostic threshold for SBP, for example, has been placed at 140 mmHg. Typically, the diagnostic threshold defines the point at which clinical intervention begins. Rose did not argue for changing the diagnostic threshold for treating disease, nor did he advocate for the use of high-cost pharmaceutical products [1]. Nevertheless, his arguments have been used to justify more aggressive treatment of CHD risk factors using expensive pharmaceutical interventions [7].

Over the course of the last decade, there have been several changes in the thresholds for clinical intervention on heart disease risk factors [8]. In this chapter and Chapters 7 and 8, we examine the rationale for these changes and estimate the impact of changing diagnostic thresholds upon a population's actual health outcomes, on the perceived health of the population, and on healthcare costs related to that population.

Definition of Health Outcomes

To state the obvious, the purpose of healthcare is to improve health. But what does this mean? We have argued that health outcomes should be defined in terms of both quantity and quality of life. A successful treatment is one that makes people live longer and/or improves quality of life [9, 10]. But there is a huge range of choices hidden in that "and/or." If we factor into the definition of disease, the distinction we have already made between true disease and pseudodisease [11], we can begin to see some constraints on the range of sensible and practical healthcare choices, but the matter of choice is still very far from simple for individual patients, for the healthcare professions, and for society in general. In this section of the chapter, we will try to take a closer look at just what desirable goals, positive health outcomes, look like. We begin by looking at how thresholds have changed.

In Chapter 5 (see especially Figs. 5.3 and 5.4, on page 000), we referred briefly to *clinical* thresholds—that is, the point at which the presence of a disease is known not because of any special screening procedure, but because observable symptoms have emerged. The appearance of very obvious symptoms of a pathology, however, is only one point on a continuum. Increasingly in modern medicine, the identification of some symptom or level of symptoms as indicative of disease depends on some threshold defined by a peer committee, and that threshold may be at some point on the continuum very far from the point defined by the clinical threshold.

Schwartz and Woloshin discussed the changes that have occurred in the diagnostic thresholds for four common health conditions [8]. In 2003, the Expert Committee on the Diagnosis and Classification of Diabetes Mellitus recommended that the threshold for diabetes be reduced from a fasting blood glucose level of 140 mg/dl down to 126 mg/dl [12]. The Joint National Committee on Detection, Evaluation, and Treatment on High Blood Pressure recommended, in 2003, that the threshold for initiation of treatment of high systolic blood pressure be moved 160 mmHg down to 140 mmHg. They also recommended that the threshold for diagnosis of elevated diastolic pressure be reduced from 100 to 90 mmHg. Following the Air Force/Texas Coronary

Table 6.1 Source and description of old and new disease definitions. (Reprinted from Schwartz and Woloshin [8], with permission from American College of Physicians.)

Disease	Source	Old definition	New Definition
Diabetes	Expert Committee on the Diagnosis and Classification of Diabetes Mellitus(7)	Fasting glucose level $\geq$ 140 mg	Fasting glucose level $\geq$ 126 mg
Hypertension (requiring treatment)	Joint National Committee on Detection Evaluation and Treatment of High Blood Pressure(8, 12)	Systolic BP $\geq$ 160 mm Hg or diastolic BP $\geq$ 100 mm Hg	Systolic BP $\geq$ 140 mm Hg or diastolic BP $\geq$90 mm Hg
Hypercholesterolemia	Air Force/Texas Coronary Atherosclerosis Prevention Study(8)	Total cholesterol level $\geq$ 240 mg	Total Cholesterol level $\geq$ 200 mg
Being overweight	National Heart, Lung, and Blood Institute(9)	Body mass index $\geq$ 27 kg/m^3	Body mass index $\geq$ 25 kg/m^3

* BP = blood pressure

Atherosclerosis Prevention Study of 1998 [13], an expert committee recommended that the threshold for high cholesterol be reduced from 240 to 200 mg/dl. Finally, the National Heart, Lung, and Blood Institute and the World Health Organization suggested that the threshold for being overweight be reduced from a body-mass index (BMI) of 27 to 25 kg/m^2. These definitions are summarized in Table 6.1.

Using data from the National Health and Nutrition Examination Survey (NHANES) Schwartz and Woloshin estimated the number of new cases of diabetes, hypertension, hypercholesterolemia, and overweight that were created by these changes in diagnostic thresholds (see Table 6.2). With a simple change in disease definition, diabetes increased 14 percent, hypertension increased 35 percent, overweight increased 42 percent, and hypercholesterolemia (high cholesterol) increased 86 percent! Under the new definitions, few people in the NHANES data set were ineligible for a chronic disease diagnosis; considering just the four conditions, three in four American adults qualified for a treatable chronic disease.

Table 6.2 Changes in prevalence of four common conditions under newly recommended definitions. (Reprinted from Schwartz and Woloshin [8], with permission from American College of physicians.)

Condition	Disease Prevalence		New Cases	Increase (%)
	Old Definition	New Definition		
Diabetes	11,897,000	13,378,000	1,681,000	14
Hypertension	38,690,000	52,100,000	13,490,000	35
Hypercholesterolemia	49,480,000	92,127,000	42,647,000	86
Being overweight	70,608,000	100,100,000	29,492,000	42
Any condition	108,750,000	140,630,000	31,880,000	29

* Numbers have been rounded to the nearest thousand. The US adult population was 187,500,000 at the time of these measurements

In the balance of this chapter, we will take a closer look at how the change in the diagnostic threshold for high blood pressure affected and is likely to affect the number of individuals diagnosed, the health status of the population, and medical care costs. In the following two chapters, we will examine the same effects created by the new definitions of high cholesterol and diabetes-overweight conditions.

What Is Blood Pressure?

Blood pressure is a measure of the adequacy of circulation. It is the balance between the blood volume ejected by the left ventricle of the heart and the resistance to blood flow in peripheral parts of the body. Adequate blood pressure is important so that the nutrients in blood can be delivered to the tissues of the body. High blood pressure causes stress on various organs and may result in stroke, diseases of the blood vessels, damage to kidneys, heart disease, and damage to the retina of the eye. On the other hand, low blood pressure, which is also associated with some risk, can cause shock, kidney failure, inadequate blood supply to the brain, and lactic acidosis. Two measures of blood pressure are commonly used in clinical settings: Systolic blood pressure (SBP) is the highest pressure during the heart's pumping cycle and is created when the left ventricle contracts. Diastolic blood pressure (DBP) is the lowest pressure during the heart's cycle. Pulse pressure is the difference between SBP and DBP. "Hypertension" is the clinical term for high blood pressure.

According to the American Heart Association defines a person who meets any one of the following four criteria is an individual with high blood pressure:

- SBP of 140 mmHg or higher, or
- DBP of 90 mmHg or higher, or
- taking antihypertensive medication, or
- being told by a physician or other healthcare provider that you have high blood pressure.

Although these definitions are commonly used in epidemiologic studies, they may lead to some inaccurate information. For example, some people who are given medication for high blood pressure may not be truly hypertensive. Others who are told by a doctor that they have high blood pressure appear not to have elevated blood pressure when examined by another doctor.

Using the American Heart Association criteria, nearly one in three adults in the USA is defined as having high blood pressure. And among this third of the general population, 30 percent do not know they have high blood pressure. Among those taking blood pressure medication, only about a third are able to bring their blood pressure into the normal range. Figure 6.2 summarizes the percent of the population with high blood pressure broken down by age and sex. From the chart, we can observe several well-established conclusions about the

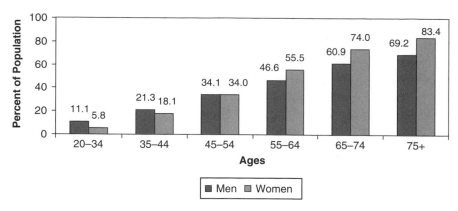

Fig. 6.2 Prevalence of high blood pressure in Americans by age and sex, NHANES: 1999–2002. (CDC/NCHS and NHLBI)

disease: High blood pressure systematically increases with age. Until age 55, more men than women have high blood pressure, but after that age the situation reverses, and high blood pressure becomes more common among women. By age 75, for example, over 83 percent of women but only 69 percent of men have high blood pressure. (For women, the risks of high blood pressure increase for those taking oral contraceptives, particularly for women who are overweight or older.)

High blood pressure is clearly a risk factor for heart attack and stroke. About half of all people who have their first heart attack and two-thirds of those who have their first stroke have blood pressures greater than 160/95 mmHg. People with SBP greater than 160 mmHg or with a DBP greater than 95 mmHg are about four times more likely to have a stroke than those with normal blood pressure. In the year 2002, high blood pressure was listed as a contributing cause of death in 261,000 cases. The statistics reported by the American Heart Association concentrate on the small portion of the population with SBPs greater than 160 mmHg or DBPs greater than 95 mmHg. According to our analysis of the National Health and Nutrition Examination Survey, only about 7.5 percent of the population has SBP greater than 160 mmHg and an even smaller percentage has DBP above 95 mmHg. Not very many people are in the extreme levels where the risk is highest. Although very high blood pressure is quite risky, there has been a growing interest in treating people who are not extreme cases.

Does Blood Pressure Treatment Save Lives?

Systematic clinical trials have clearly demonstrated that blood pressure treatment is valuable for people with hypertension. These clinical trials have shown that antihypertensive therapy may lower the number of new strokes by

35–40 percent. In addition, heart attacks might be reduced by 20–25 percent. Heart failure is the clinical term for weakening of the heart pump function. Inadequate pumping of blood by the heart often results in the accumulation of fluids in blood vessels. Some of the biggest benefits of blood pressure management are for heart failure, where appropriate management might reduce new cases by 50 percent. For people with established high blood pressure, or for people with heart failure, the benefits of treatment seem quite clear.

On the other hand, we know very little about the benefits of lowering the blood pressure for those whose blood pressure is only a little bit high. The problem is that there are very few systematic studies of drug treatment for people with normal blood pressure. It is often assumed that if someone has an SBP of 140 mmHg and it is lowered to 120 mmHg, then the person would reduce his or her risks to the level corresponding to his or her newly lower blood pressure. In other words, if one lowered one's blood pressure to 120 mmHg then one would have the same risk as people who are already at 120 mmHg. However, studies do not show this level of benefit. In the Hypertension Detection and Follow-up Program (HDFP), the risks appear to be intermediate between the starting level and the ending level [14]. In other words, a person who lowered his SBP from 140 to 120 mmHg would achieve about the same risk level as someone at 130 mmHg.

High blood pressure is a serious health problem—no reasonable person would deny that. But newer definitions of high blood pressure concentrate on people with less extreme blood pressure readings. This is most clearly described in the 7th Joint National Commission on High Blood Pressure report, discussed in the next section of this chapter, where we show why the downward shift in what constitutes high blood pressure *are* controversial.

Review of Controversies

According to a variety of data sets, about 24 percent of the adult population have prevalent hypertension under the current definition as SBP > 140 or DBP > 90 mmHg [15]. Using population surveys, the proportion of the population with hypertension has remained stable over the last 40 years. However, even before the change in the diagnostic threshold for high blood pressure, the proportion of the population diagnosed and treated for hypertension has systematically increased [16]. Between 1970 and 2000, the proportion of the population aware that it had hypertension, the proportion treated for high blood pressure, and the proportion with controlled blood pressure systematically increased [17]. Changing the diagnostic threshold for hypertension from 160/95 to 140/90 approximately doubled the number of cases [16].

It might appear that the change in diagnostic threshold with more aggressive management of hypertension has produced positive results. For example, MacMahon and colleagues pooled the results from seven observational studies with stroke outcomes and nine observational studies on CHD outcomes. The relative risk of stroke began to increase systematically with DBPs exceeding 91 mmHg. Those with DBP readings of 105 mmHg were nearly 3.5 times more likely to experience stroke than those with DBP values of 90 mmHg or lower. Similarly, the risks for CHD increased to over 2.0 for those with DBP of 105 mmHg or higher [18]. The Joint National Commission on high blood pressure noted that aggressive treatment of high blood pressure coincided with significant declines in stroke between 1960 and 1990 [19].

Unfortunately, the evidence about the effectiveness of aggressive management of high blood pressure is not so clear. For example, the decrease in strokes exceeds what would be expected given studies on the effect of blood pressure control. One analysis pooled results from nine clinical trials and noted that a 5.6-mmHg decrease in DBP was associated with a 38-percent decrease in stroke. Yet, between 1970 and 1980, there was about a 1-mmHg decline in DBP. During that period, the actual observed decline in stroke was 43 percent. Best estimates based on the relationship between blood pressure and stroke suggest that the reduction should have been only about 18 percent [20]. Similarly, the Minnesota Heart Study showed significant annual declines in stroke over the course of time, but the decline was uncorrelated with hypertension in their population [21]. So, it remains unclear whether the decline in stroke is associated with better control of blood pressure.

When making comparisons between different populations, epidemiologists use standard age corrections because blood pressure tends to increase with advancing age. These methods allow us to compare people who are at equivalent ages. The American Heart Association emphasizes that there has been a recent increase in the age-adjusted death rate from high blood pressure. They note that between 1992 and 2002, this rate jumped by over 25 percent, and that the actual number of deaths attributed to high blood pressure increased by 50 percent. However, the general trend has gone in the other direction. The NHANES has been conducted three times. It was first completed between 1976 and 1980. The second survey was completed between 1988 and 1994, and the third between 1999 and 2002. Figure 6.3 shows the prevalence of high blood pressure broken down by race/ethnicity and sex. It is true that there was a slight increase in the proportion of the population with high blood pressure between the 1988–94 and the 1999–02 surveys. This happened in all groups except Mexican-American men. However, considering the long-haul of 26 years, the studies showed a significant decline in the proportion of the population with high blood pressure between the first and the second surveys. In the interval between 1976 and 1988, the crisis of high blood pressure appeared to be getting better rather than worse. In other words, the market for the treatment of high blood pressure was declining rather than expanding. The American Heart Association tends to focus on the relatively weak data that support their point and to ignore the relatively stronger trend that has emerged over the last several decades. Some believe that there is pressure to diagnose more people with high blood pressure as a way to increase the number of people being

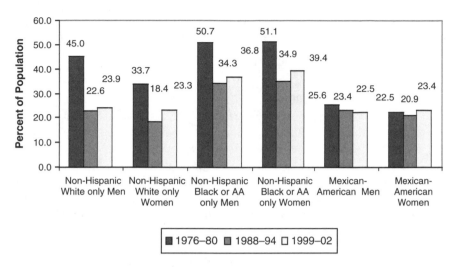

Fig. 6.3 Age-Adjusted prevalence trends for high blood pressure in Americans age 20–74 by Race/Ethnicity, sex and Survey, NHAWES: 1976–80, 1988–94, and 1999–2002. (From AHA 2005.) (CDC/NCHS. Data based on a single measure of BP.)

treated. One way to expand the market for hypertension treatment is to change the definition of high blood pressure.

In summary, there has been a recent reduction in the rate of heart attack and stroke in the population. There have also been aggressive efforts to control blood pressure. Although control of blood pressure is very likely to have contributed to the reduction in heart attacks and strokes, the pattern of outcomes does not clearly fit the data. For example, the average blood pressure in the population went down between about 1976 and 1994. During that same period, the rates of death from heart attacks and strokes also went down. So, it looked like the declining blood pressures may have been associated with declining death rates. However, over the last decade, the average blood pressures have been rising while the rate of premature death from heart disease and stroke continues to fall. At least at the population level, the relationship between blood pressure and heart attacks may be weaker than it appears on the surface. At the individual level, the risks of very high blood pressure are clearly established. For people with only modestly elevated blood pressure, the data fit less clearly. Some studies suggest that other factors may have an important impact on the number of strokes experienced by people in the population.

JNC-7

The National Heart Lung and Blood Institute (NHLBI) has administered the National High Blood Pressure Education Program (NHBPEP) for over three decades. In May 2003, the commission released its seventh national report, known as JNC-7 [22]. Successive JNC reports have pushed for lower diagnostic thresholds for high blood pressure. JNC-6 defined high-normal blood pressure as SBP = 130–139 mmHg and DBP = 85–89 mmHg. JNC-7 goes a step further by defining a new condition known as prehypertension. Individuals in this category have an SBP of 120–139 mmHg or a DBP of 80–89 mmHg [22]. For people aged 50 or over, nearly 40 percent will fall into the prehypertensive or hypertensive categories. Although many people will be labeled as prehypertensive, the report does not suggest the use of antihypertensive drugs in this category. Instead, behavioral intervention is indicated. On the surface, the rationale for creating the new category of prehypertension is compelling. Epidemiologic studies of adults between the ages of 40 and 70 suggest that each increase in SBP of 20 mmHg and each increase in DBP of 10 mmHg results in a doubling of CVD risk except for those with blood pressures lower than 115/75 mmHg [23]. The report argued that management of blood pressure using medication results in a 40-percent reduction in the incidence of stroke, a 25-percent reduction in the incidence of MI, and a 50-percent reduction in the incidence of heart failure [24]. However, large clinical trials have not shown benefits for lowering high-normal to optimal blood pressure [25]. Furthermore, it is unclear what benefit to expect from lifestyle intervention among those in the prehypertension range.

Justification for Lowering the Threshold

The rationale for the JNC-7 recommendation to lower diagnostic thresholds was that people with moderately high blood pressure are at increased risk for heart attack and stroke just as those with very high blood pressure are at risk. The argument was based on a comprehensive review of the research literature. However, the most important piece of evidence came from the Prospective Studies Collaborative. This group summarized 61 other studies involving more than 1 million adults. They used a technique known as meta-analysis, which sums together the observations from all the different studies. The results of the meta-analysis are presented in Fig. 6.4. The graph shows the relationship between SBP and stroke and the relationship between DBP and stroke. The four lines on the left and right of the figure are for different age groups. There appears to be a strong positive correlation between blood pressure and stroke. For the DBP, for example, it would appear that the benefit one gains from reducing blood pressure by 5 mmHg is the same for people whose initial values are very high (let us call them "high starters," with DBP readings over 100 mmHg), and for those who are initially low ("low starters," with readings 75 mmHg). Thus, it would seem that reducing the threshold for high DBP is a wise thing to do across the board—the benefit appears to be equal for low starters and high starters, but many more people will be helped because many

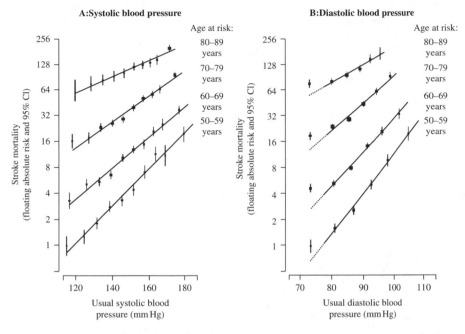

Fig. 6.4 Blood pressure and the risk of stroke. From prospective studies collaboration-61 studies, 1 million adults. (Reprinted from Olsen and Gøtzsche [26], with permission from Elsevier.)

more low starters will be getting treatment. And in fact, investing in blood pressure reduction for people with relatively low blood pressure might ultimately be a good use of resources. This would be perfectly consistent with the ideas proposed by Geoffrey Rose.

Although the Prospective Studies Collaborative suggests a linear relationship between blood pressure and stroke, it is important to examine Fig. 6.4 in more detail. Two features are important. First, values closer to normal are actually off the diagonal. Look at the points on the graph above diastolic pressures of 70 mmHg. In each case, they are not on the line, but rather higher. Second, and the most important feature of Fig. 6.4, is that the y-axis is not a linear scale. Instead, it is a base-2 logarithmic scale. The relationship between blood pressure and stroke is not linear. It is log-linear. That means that each point on the y-axis is twice as large as the preceding point, while the x-axis increases in a linear fashion, at set increments of 20 mmHg.

In order to gain a better understanding of the relationships, we redrew the SBP portion of Fig. 6.4. The revised graph is shown as Fig. 6.5. The difference between the two graphs is that the latter uses ordinary units on the y-axis. The most striking feature in Fig. 6.5 is that there is an inflection point at about 150 mmHg. This is the point at which the probability of stroke quite suddenly becomes much higher. By comparison, the suddenness of this change is not so

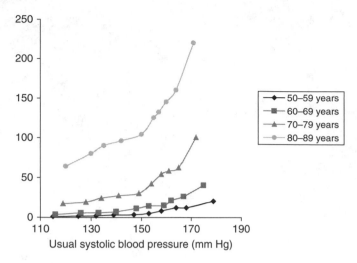

Fig. 6.5 Data from the Prospective Studies Collaboration (Fig. 6.4) with linear units for stoke mortality on the y-axis (Adapted from Kaplan & Ong [25])

easy to see in Fig. 6.4. For the lower age groups in Fig. 6.5, the relationship between SBP and stroke is quite flat up to above 140 mmHg. These results are consistent with most previously published articles in the literature. In other words, the probability of having a stroke is not linearly related to blood pressure. In fact, the previous (unrevised) thresholds for initiation of treatment—at 140 mmHg for SBP—appear to have a clear rationale. (And, as it turns out, the same is true for the unrevised threshold for initiation of treatment for diastolic pressure—90 mmHg also appears to be the right number.)

Of course, there may be some very slight benefit in initiating treatment for those who have DBP below 140 mmHg. After all, in the two older groups especially, the curves do not go from *flat* to steep at the inflection point; the change is more like going from a slow increase to a fast increase. But the question remains, should individuals with a DBP of less than 140 mmHg expose themselves to medications that have side effects, and should they endure the expense? Nonpharmacological treatments, such as diet and exercise, may be of great value. Moreover, those prescribed medication may be less motivated to change their lifestyles.

One concern about the treatment of people with mild hypertension (SBP 120–140 mmHg or DPB 80–90 mmHg) is that few clinical trials have evaluated people who have prehypertension but do not have other risk factors. Table 6.3 summarizes a sampling of studies that have often been cited as supporting aggressive management of blood pressure. The few studies that included participants with relatively normal blood pressure focused on patients with other CHD risk factors, including established coronary disease, diabetes mellitus, and renal disease. The third column labeled "Predominant risk factor" is particularly important. There appear to be few studies of people in the prehypertensive

Table 6.3 Characteristics of participants in selected studies of hypertension treatment

Study	Sample Size	Predominant risk factor	BP at baseline
Hypertension Detection and Follow-up Program [14]	10,940	Hypertensive, but not on medication	All DBPs >90 and <104 mmHg
Prospective Randomized trial—Vascular Effects of Norvasc Trial (PRE-VENT) [27]	825	History of CV complications	129/79 mmHg (34% measured while on medication)
African American Study of Kidney Disease and Hypertension (AASK) [28]	1,094 (all African-American, ages 18–70)	1,094 hypertensive patients who also had renal disease	150/95 mmHg
Irbesartan Diabetic Nephropathy Trial LIFE [29]	9,193	Hypertensive patients with nephropathy due to Type 2 diabetes	174/98 mmHg
Appropriate Blood Pressure Control in Diabetes Trial (ABCD) [30]	480	All subjects had diabetes mellitus	136/84 mmHg
Diabetes, hypertension, microalbuminuria or proteinuria, cardiovascular events, and ramipril (DIABHYCAR) [31, 32]	4,912	All subjects had diabetes mellitus	146/83 mmHg
Hypertension in the Very Elderly Trial (HYVET) [33]	1,283 (all elderly)	Previous hypertension	181/100
The Irbesartan Type II Diabetic Nephropathy Trial (IDNT2) [34, 35]	1,715	All subjects had diabetes mellitus and renal disease	159/87
NIsoldipine in Coronary artery disease in LEuven (NICOLE) [36]	819	All subjects had established coronary disease and underwent PTCA	129/78
Treatment of Mild Hypertension Study (TOMHS) [37]	844	All subjects had mild hypertension, defined as DBP 90–99 mmHg without medication, or 85–99 mmHg if using medications	140/91
Trial of Preventing Hypertension (TROPHY) [38]	772	56% had total cholesterol values >200 mg/dl, 38% had triglycerides 150 mg/dl	134/84

range without other risk factors. The one exception is the Trial of Preventing Hypertension (TROPHY) [38]. In this study, 409 adults with SBP between 130 and 139 mmHg and DBP < 89 mmHg or DBP between 85 and 89 mmHg and SBP < 139 mmHg were randomly assigned to an angiotensin-receptor blocker (ARB) or to a placebo. The placebo group was significantly more likely to progress to hypertension and to experience serious adverse events over the next 4 years.

Progression from pre-hypertension to actual hypertension has been investigated in the Framingham cohort for different age groups (35–64 and 65–94) [39]. After adjusting for sex, age, BMI, baseline examinations, and baseline SBP and DBP, individuals with SBPs between 130 and 139 or DBPs between 85 and 89 progressed to hypertension after 4 years in 37.3 percent of those aged 35–64 and 49.5 percent of those aged 65–94. Individuals with SBPs between 120 and 129 or DBPs between 80 and 84 progressed to hypertension after 4 years in 17.6 percent of those aged 35 and 64 and 25.5 percent of those aged 65 and 94. Of note, 20 and 30 percent of individuals with blood pressure in the "prehypertension" range spontaneously reduced their blood pressure to normal.

It is interesting to consider the results of the TROPHY clinical trial in light of these observational data. In the TROPHY trial, the rate of progression from prehypertension to hypertension was significantly higher in the placebo group (63 percent) than would be expected based on observational data. The rate of progression in the treated group (53 percent) is closer to what observational studies would suggest [38]. Another concern about the TROPHY study is that changes in blood pressure were relatively modest. The initial decrease in blood pressure was less than 10 mmHg of diastolic pressure and 5 mmHg of diastolic pressure. However, after the treatment stopped, 24 months into the study, placebo and active treatment groups were virtually the same (they differed by only about 2 mmHg).

ARBs, the drug used in TROPHY, are not the recommended first-line treatment for managing blood pressure. JNC-7 suggests the use of cheaper medications that have a longer history of efficacy and safety. (Diuretics top the list.) However, diuretics and other cheap and time-tested drugs are not profitable for pharmaceutical companies. Presumably, the selection of ARBs by the TROPHY investigators was because these medications have the longest future patent protection. Although ARBs work through a similar mechanism to the well-regarded angiotensin-concerting enzyme (ACE) inhibitors, not all investigators believe they are as safe. Some evidence suggests that ARBs increase the risk of heart attacks [40].

Likelihood of Benefit–Chances of Side Effects

No treatment is completely without side effects, some of which are risky. When there are such side effects, patients must decide if they are willing to expose themselves to the risks. Glasziou and Irwig [41] have analyzed this problem and

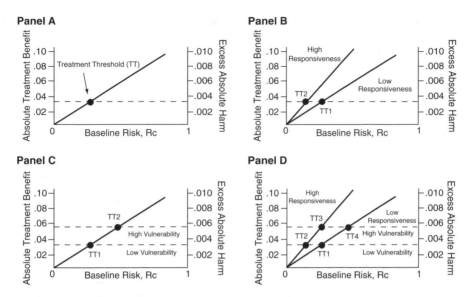

Fig. 6.6 The solid line in panel *A* shows the relationship between the benefits of treatment and the risks of the illness. The dashed line shows the chances of harm due to side effects of treatment. The point where the lines intersect is the treatment threshold, or the point at which treatment should be considered. Panels B, C, and D outline other situations. Panel B shows that the treatment threshold should be lower for high responders than for low responders. The different horizontal dashed lines in Panel C indicate patients who are sensitive to medication and highly vulnerable to side effects. Panel D shows treatment thresholds for different combinations or response to treatment and vulnerability to side effects (Reprinted from Kravitz et al. [42] with permission from Wiley-Blackwell.)

concluded that the benefits of treatment go disproportionately to patients who are most seriously affected by the disease. The risk of side effects may be worth it for someone who without treatment is at risk of dying or becoming disabled by a disease.

Similarly, the lower the risk of the disease, the lower the benefit of treatment. Figure 6.6 provides a pictorial explanation of their ideas. Consider Panel A in the figure. The solid line shows the relationship between the benefits of treatment and the risks of the illness. In this case, imagine the risk factor is blood pressure and the outcome is stroke. As blood pressure increases, the chances of stroke also increase. The dashed line shows the chances of harm due to side effects of treatment. Everyone exposed to the treatment experiences these consequences, and they are independent of the level of risk. The point where the lines intersect is the "treatment threshold," or the point at which treatment should be considered.

Panels B, C, and D in Fig. 6.6 outline other situations. Not all people respond to treatment the same way. Some are very responsive to treatment (high responders) and others are less responsive (low responders). Panel B shows that the treatment threshold (TT2) should be lower for high responders. Similarly, some people are more sensitive to the medication and are highly vulnerable to side effects. Others may have low vulnerability. These are indicated by different horizontal dashed lines in Panel C. It shows that the treatment threshold TT2 should be higher for those who are more vulnerable to side effects. Panel D shows treatment thresholds for different combinations or responses to treatment and vulnerability to side effects (figure from Kravitz, Duan, & Braslow [42]).

How Many People Will be Affected by the New Guidelines?

Using simulation techniques, we estimated the impact of lowering blood pressure diagnostic thresholds upon a population's health status. A variety of assumptions were used to create these models. First, the population distribution of blood pressure was estimated using data from the Third NHANES (NHANES III). NHANES III was conducted between 1988 and 1994 by the National Center for Health Statistics of the Centers for Disease Control and Prevention (CDC). The purpose of the survey was to evaluate the health and nutritional status of the civilian non-institutionalized population of the USA. The study uses a national sample of approximately 34,000 people 2 months of age or older. In addition to household interviews, 73 percent of the sample had blood drawn and underwent physical examination. Our analysis will focus on approximately 20,000 men and women aged 17 or older for whom physical examination data were available. The data set is available from the National Center for Health Statistics at the following site: www.cdc.gov/nchswww/mchshome.htm

Analysis of the data requires weighting by primary sampling unit (PSU) to account for the complicated multi-staged sampling. Guidelines for the analysis of NHANES data were summarized by Schwartz and Woloshin [43].

Figure 6.7 shows the distribution of SBP in the US population. This distribution is relatively normal. Very few people have SBPs of less than 90 mmHg. Similarly, very few people have SBPs greater than 160 mmHg. Most people fall toward the middle. As we move left on the graph from 160 down toward the center of the distribution, more and more people are picked up. As you can see, the portion of the population falling above 120 mmHg is very large. In other words, changing the definition also substantially changes the number of people eligible for treatment. To put it another way, the "eligible for treatment" number goes from a small percentage of the population to a very large percentage.

Using data from the NHANES, we estimated that about 4 percent of the population is in the highest risk category, with SBPs greater than 160 mmHg. These are the people who are at high risk for stroke or heart attack. About

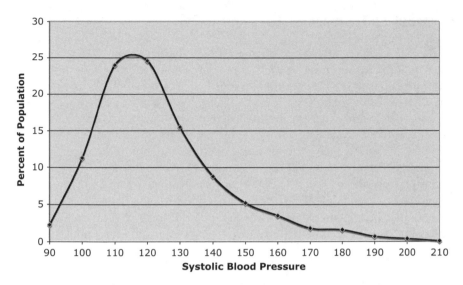

Fig. 6.7 Distribution of systolic blood pressure from the NHANES III

14 percent have SBPs greater than 140 mmHg. However, using the new definition of prehypertension, nearly 40 percent qualify for a diagnosis. Furthermore, this number goes up systematically with age. For older adults, the great majority of the population are eligible for the diagnosis if the new definitions are used. If we apply the criteria of current medication use, or SBP > 120 mmHg, or DBP > 90 mmHg, more than 90 percent of those over 65 should be on treatment. Once diagnosed, it remains unclear whether treatment will be valuable. Those with prehypertension may benefit from treatment, but they must also face the medical consequences and the costs of treatment. For these people, the potential gains are much smaller than for those with very high blood pressure, but the consequences of treatment are about the same. In other words, those with near-normal blood pressure take similar risks when they use medication, but gain much less potential benefit.

In summary, changes in the diagnostic threshold for high blood pressure have led to the identification of 13 million new cases. The new category of prehypertension will include up to 40 percent of the population and up to 90 percent of adults 60 years of age or older. The consequences of high blood pressure, including stroke and CHD, have been systematically declining, and it would appear the changes in diagnostic thresholds have resulted in better population health. However, the observed decline in stroke and CHD has been much more rapid than would be expected from changes in blood pressure as actually measured in the population.

Paradoxical Treatment Effects

The decision to include the new category of prehypertension in JNC 7 was based on an analysis of the Framingham Heart Study demonstrating that adults with blood pressures in the 125/80–130/89 range had an increased risk, as compared with those with normal blood pressure, of progression to hypertension [39]. This was particularly true for those participants who were 65 years or older at baseline. However, when we examined the paper, we noted that for adults less than 65 years of age, the probability of transition from optimum blood pressure (defined as SBP < 130 and DPB < 85 mmHg) to hypertension over a 4-year interval is only about 5 percent. The transition from normal blood pressure to hypertension is about 18 percent over this 4-year interval. It was clear from the analysis that older individuals with normal blood pressure (now called prehypertension) were more likely to progress to hypertension than younger adults. However, it is not entirely clear that treatment of older adults offers the same benefits as treatment of younger adults.

For older adults, some paradoxical effects of treatment have been reported in the literature. Substantial evidence suggests that blood pressure, blood cholesterol, and blood glucose all increase with age [17]. However, the meaning of elevated CHD risk factors for the elderly is less clear. Several studies have failed to show that elevated blood pressure is a predictor of mortality for the elderly [21]. One unexpected finding was reported in a community-based study in Finland, in which investigators found that elevated SBP and DBP predicted *survival* rather than death in women and men who were 85 years and older [44].

Langer, Ganiats, and Barrett-Connor confirmed the Finnish finding DBP in men 75 years and older [45, 46]. Using data from an epidemiologic study in Rancho Bernardo, CA, they found that the risk of cardiovascular death for older men declines with increasing blood pressure. As expected, higher levels of DBP are associated with higher probabilities of death for younger men. These findings were unaffected by statistical adjustments for body mass, elevated cholesterol, high-density lipoprotein cholesterol, fasting blood glucose, pulse pressure, and cigarette smoking. Including suggested paradoxical effects in sensitivity analysis will further broaden our evaluation of policy options

Using data from the Prospective Studies Collaboration, we estimated the change in the absolute risk of developing a stroke for someone aged 60–69. The analysis suggests that the absolute risk reduction would decline from about 0.7 percent (seven-tenths of one percentage point) to about 0.5 percent (one-fifth of a percentage point). In other words, a 60-year-old with a DBP of 90 mmHg will have a 99.3 percent chance of being stroke-free for the next 10 years. Taking the effort to reduce DBP to 80 mmHg improves absolute risk of avoiding a stroke to about 99.5 percent. Is it worth it?

Conclusions

It has been more than a 15 years since the publication of Geoffrey Rose's epic monograph "The Strategy of Preventive Medicine." Rose argued that we must be more aggressive in bringing prevention to the masses. Changes in the population distribution for risk factors can have substantial effects on population health. Rose's arguments have been used to stimulate more aggressive intervention for individuals previously thought not to need treatment. However, Rose's arguments may have been misused. He favored aggressive intervention using behavioral and public-health methods that were low cost. Instead, we have seen greater use of aggressive screening and intervention with high-cost pharmaceutical products.

This chapter explored the implications of changing the definitions of high blood pressure. The most dramatic single instance of a change in definitions came about in 2003, with the release of JNC-7 and the creation of a new category known as prehypertension. Individuals previously categorized as normal now qualify for this new diagnosis. Analysis of the NHANES shows that the change of definition has had profound effects on the number of people who might be labeled as having a blood pressure problem. In the adult population, the number of people affected would go from about 14 percent to about 40 percent. In other words, there would be a 185-percent increase. We do not know how many people would seek or gain treatment for prehypertension or whether the treatment would be effective. Clinical trials have not evaluated pharmaceutical interventions for people who were previously thought to have normal blood pressure. Using observational data, it appears that the benefit of treatment will be quite small. On the other hand, the costs of the treatment are likely to be substantial.

New pharmacological approaches to the treatment of high blood pressure are very expensive, costing as much as several dollars per day. For a 50-year-old diagnosed with prehypertension, the drug cost might be $500 or more per year, and this cost would be incurred each year for the remainder of his lifespan. In addition, there are substantial monitoring costs because people taking medications need to visit their physicians more often. The cost would be high and the benefits would be uncertain.

The Joint National Commission on high blood pressure does not recommend pharmacological therapy for prehypertension. Like Geoffry Rose, they suggest lifestyle modification. Nevertheless, we know that lifestyle modification is rarely used or promoted by physicians.

In sum, there has been a trend toward the expansion of the market for hypertension treatments. These treatments are very effective for people with serious high blood pressure. Treatment effect for people with near-normal blood pressure is less well understood. However, we do know that the broadened market for these medicines will lead to substantial profits for pharmaceutical companies. The expansion of the drug market is not unique to high blood pressure medications. In the next few chapters, we will look at similar problems in the management of high blood cholesterol, high blood sugar, and overweight.

References

1. Rose GA. *The Strategy of Preventive Medicine*. Oxford England; New York: Oxford University Press; 1992.
2. Goldstein LB, Adams R, Becker K, et al. Primary prevention of ischemic stroke: A statement for healthcare professionals from the Stroke Council of the American Heart Association. *Stroke*. Jan 2001;32(1):280–299.
3. Howard G, Howard VJ. Ethnic disparities in stroke: the scope of the problem. *Ethn Dis*. Fall 2001;11(4):761–768.
4. MRC/BHF Heart Protection Study of cholesterol lowering with simvastatin in 20,536 high-risk individuals: a randomised placebo-controlled trial. *Lancet*. Jul 6 2002; 360(9326):7–22.
5. Marmot MG, Poulter NR. Primary prevention of stroke. *Lancet*. Feb 8 1992; 339(8789): 344–347.
6. Rose G, Day S. The population mean predicts the number of deviant individuals. *BMJ*. Nov 3 1990;301(6759):1031–1034.
7. Summary of the second report of the National Cholesterol Education Program (NCEP) Expert Panel on Detection, Evaluation, and Treatment of High Blood Cholesterol in Adults (Adult Treatment Panel II). *JAMA*. Jun 16 1993;269(23):3015–3023.
8. Schwartz LM, Woloshin S. Changing disease definitions: implications for disease prevalence. Analysis of the Third National Health and Nutrition Examination Survey, 1988–1994. *Eff Clin Pract*. Mar–Apr 1999;2(2):76–85.
9. Kaplan RM, Wingard DL. Trends in breast cancer incidence, survival, and mortality. *Lancet*. Aug 12 2000;356(9229):592–593.
10. Kaplan RM. The Ziggy Theorem – toward an outcomes-focused health psychology. *Health Psychol*. 1994;13(6):451–460.
11. Black WC, Welch HG. Screening for disease. *AJR Am J Roentgenol*. 1997;168(1):3–11.
12. Report of the Expert Committee on the Diagnosis and Classification of Diabetes Mellitus. *Diabetes Care*. Jul 1997;20(7):1183–1197.
13. Downs JR, Clearfield M, Weis S, et al. Primary prevention of acute coronary events with lovastatin in men and women with average cholesterol levels: results of AFCAPS/ TexCAPS. Air Force/Texas Coronary Atherosclerosis Prevention Study. *JAMA*. 1998; 279(20):1615–1622.
14. Persistence of reduction in blood pressure and mortality of participants in the Hypertension Detection and Follow-up Program. Hypertension Detection and Follow-up Program Cooperative Group. *JAMA*. Apr 8 1988;259(14):2113–2122.
15. Burt VL, Whelton P, Roccella EJ, et al. Prevalence of hypertension in the US adult population. Results from the Third National Health and Nutrition Examination Survey, 1988–1991. *Hypertension*. Mar 1995;25(3):305–313.
16. Vallbona C, Pavlik V. Advances in the community control of hypertension: from epidemiology to primary care practice. *J Hypertens Suppl*. Dec 1992;10(7):S51–57.
17. Whelton PK, He J, Appel LJ, et al. Primary prevention of hypertension: clinical and public health advisory from The National High Blood Pressure Education Program. *JAMA*. Oct 16 2002;288(15):1882–1888.
18. MacMahon S. Antihypertensive drug treatment: the potential, expected and observed effects on vascular disease. *J Hypertens Suppl*. Dec 1990;8(7):S239–244.

19. The fifth report of the Joint National Committee on Detection, Evaluation, and Treatment of High Blood Pressure (JNC V). *Arch Intern Med.* Jan 25 1993;153(2):154–183.

20. Langer RD. The epidemiology of hypertension control in populations. *Clin Exp Hypertens.* Oct 1995;17(7):1127–1144.

21. Luepker RV, Jacobs DR, Jr., Folsom AR, et al. Cardiovascular risk factor change–1973-74 to 1980-82: the Minnesota Heart Survey. *J Clin Epidemiol.* 1988;41(9):825–833.

22. Chobanian AV, Bakris GL, Black HR, et al. The Seventh Report of the Joint National Committee on Prevention, Detection, Evaluation, and Treatment of High Blood Pressure: the JNC 7 report. *JAMA.* May 21 2003;289(19):2560–2572.

23. Lewington S, Clarke R, Qizilbash N, Peto R, Collins R. Age-specific relevance of usual blood pressure to vascular mortality: a meta-analysis of individual data for one million adults in 61 prospective studies. *Lancet.* Dec 14 2002;360(9349):1903–1913.

24. Neal B, MacMahon S, Chapman N. Effects of ACE inhibitors, calcium antagonists, and other blood-pressure-lowering drugs: results of prospectively designed overviews of randomised trials. Blood Pressure Lowering Treatment Trialists' Collaboration. *Lancet.* Dec 9 2000;356(9246):1955–1964.

25. Kaplan RM, Ong M. Rationale and Public Health Implications of Changing CHD Risk Factor Definitions. *Annu Rev Public Health.* 2007;28:321–344.

26. Olsen O, Gøtzsche PC. Cochrane review on screen for breast cancer with mammography. *The Lancet.* 2001;358(9290).

27. Byington RP, Miller ME, Herrington D, et al. Rationale, design, and baseline characteristics of the Prospective Randomized Evaluation of the Vascular Effects of Norvasc Trial (PREVENT). *Am J Cardiol.* Oct 15 1997;80(8):1087–1090.

28. Wright JT, Jr., Bakris G, Greene T, et al. Effect of blood pressure lowering and antihypertensive drug class on progression of hypertensive kidney disease: results from the AASK trial. *JAMA.* Nov 20 2002;288(19):2421–2431.

29. Lewis EJ, Hunsicker LG, Clarke WR, et al. Renoprotective effect of the angiotensin-receptor antagonist irbesartan in patients with nephropathy due to Type 2 diabetes. *N Engl J Med.* Sep 20 2001;345(12):851–860.

30. Estacio RO, Savage S, Nagel NJ, Schrier RW. Baseline characteristics of participants in the Appropriate Blood Pressure Control in Diabetes trial. *Control Clin Trials.* Jun 1996;17(3):242–257.

31. Lievre M, Marre M, Chatellier G, et al. The non-insulin-dependent diabetes, hypertension, microalbuminuria or proteinuria, cardiovascular events, and ramipril (DIABHYCAR) study: design, organization, and patient recruitment. DIABHYCAR Study Group. *Control Clin Trials.* Aug 2000;21(4):383–396.

32. Marre M, Lievre M, Chatellier G, Mann JF, Passa P, Menard J. Effects of low dose ramipril on cardiovascular and renal outcomes in patients with Type 2 diabetes and raised excretion of urinary albumin: randomised, double blind, placebo controlled trial (the DIABHYCAR study). *BMJ.* Feb 28 2004;328(7438):495.

33. Bulpitt C, Fletcher A, Beckett N, et al. Hypertension in the very elderly trial (HYVET): protocol for the main trial. *Drugs Aging.* 2001;18(3):151–164.

34. Pohl MA, Blumenthal S, Cordonnier DJ, et al. Independent and additive impact of blood pressure control and angiotensin II receptor blockade on renal outcomes in the irbesartan diabetic nephropathy trial: clinical implications and limitations. *J Am Soc Nephrol.* Oct 2005;16(10):3027–3037.

35. Rodby RA, Rohde RD, Clarke WR, et al. The Irbesartan Type II diabetic nephropathy trial: study design and baseline patient characteristics. For the Collaborative Study Group. *Nephrol Dial Transplant.* Apr 2000;15(4):487–497.

36. Dens JA, Desmet WJ, Coussement P, et al. Usefulness of Nisoldipine for prevention of restenosis after percutaneous transluminal coronary angioplasty (results of the NICOLE study). NIsoldipine in COronary artery disease in LEuven. *Am J Cardiol.* Jan 1 2001;87(1):28–33.

37. Liebson PR, Grandits GA, Dianzumba S, et al. Comparison of five antihypertensive monotherapies and placebo for change in left ventricular mass in patients receiving nutritional-hygienic therapy in the Treatment of Mild Hypertension Study (TOMHS). *Circulation*. Feb 1 1995;91(3):698–706.
38. Julius S, Nesbitt SD, Egan BM, et al. Feasibility of treating prehypertension with an angiotensin-receptor blocker. *N Engl J Med*. Apr 20 2006;354(16):1685–1697.
39. Vasan RS, Larson MG, Leip EP, Kannel WB, Levy D. Assessment of frequency of progression to hypertension in non-hypertensive participants in the Framingham Heart Study: a cohort study. *Lancet*. Nov 17 2001;358(9294):1682–1686.
40. Strauss MH, Hall AS. Angiotensin receptor blockers may increase risk of myocardial infarction: unraveling the ARB-MI paradox. *Circulation*. Aug 22 2006;114(8):838–854.
41. Glasziou PP, Irwig LM. An evidence based approach to individualising treatment. *BMJ*. Nov 18 1995;311(7016):1356–1359.
42. Kravitz RL, Duan N, Braslow J. Evidence-based medicine, heterogeneity of treatment effects, and the trouble with averages. *Milbank Q*. 2004;82(4):661–687.
43. Schwartz LM, Woloshin S. Changing disease definitions: implications for disease prevalence. Analysis of the Third National Health and Nutrition Examination Survey, 1988–1994. *Eff Clin Pract*. 1999;2(2):76–85.
44. Mattila K, Haavisto M, Rajala S, Heikinheimo R. Blood pressure and five year survival in the very old. *Br Med J (Clin Res Ed)*. Mar 26 1988;296(6626):887–889.
45. Langer RD, Ganiats TG, Barrett-Connor E. Factors associated with paradoxical survival at higher blood pressures in the very old. *Am J Epidemiol*. Jul 1 1991;134(1):29–38.
46. Langer RD, Ganiats TG, Barrett-Connor E. Paradoxical survival of elderly men with high blood pressure. *BMJ*. May 20 1989;298(6684):1356–1357.

Chapter 7
The Cholesterol Cutoff

Recently, while changing clothes after a workout in the gym, I could not resist listening in as two men exchanged numbers in what sounded like a boasting fest. Was it about their golf scores or some other index of athletic accomplishment? Were they comparing earnings on their stock portfolios or citing the IQ scores of their children? No. They were talking about their serum cholesterol readings. A low cholesterol value is not only a number people know, it is also a source of pride. One man had lowered his LDL cholesterol through vigorous exercise and the use of medication. He attributed his regular visits to the gym as part of this quest. This chapter explores the benefits and other consequences of our obsession with cholesterol.

Cholesterol is a waxy substance found in the cell walls of most animals. It is necessary for a variety of reasons, including the production of sexual and other hormones and building and maintaining cell membranes. It is not an exaggeration to say that cholesterol is essential to life. However, excessive levels are dangerous because high cholesterol may increase the risk for heart disease. The term "hypercholesterolemia" is used to describe abnormally high levels of cholesterol in the blood. There is no doubt that hypercholesterolemia is one of the strongest risk factors for the development of CVD. The amount of research evidence is simply overwhelming.

Evidence for the relationship between cholesterol and heart disease has been accumulating for more than 50 years. One of the best-known research projects to establish that relationship was the Seven Countries Study, which began in the 1950s. In this investigation, middle-aged men from Japan, Greece, Yugoslavia, Italy, The Netherlands, The USA, and Finland had their blood cholesterol measured. Over the course of years, the population was followed for death from heart disease or for the development of heart attacks. Countries that had the highest cholesterol levels also had the highest rates of CVD (see Fig. 7.1) [1]. However, though the study showed a strong correlation between blood cholesterol and heart disease, it did not prove a causal relationship. In other words, it demonstrated that those with high levels of cholesterol were more likely to develop heart disease, but it left unanswered the question of whether lowering cholesterol would lower heart disease.

R.M. Kaplan, *Disease, Diagnoses, and Dollars*, DOI 10.1007/978-0-387-74045-4_7,

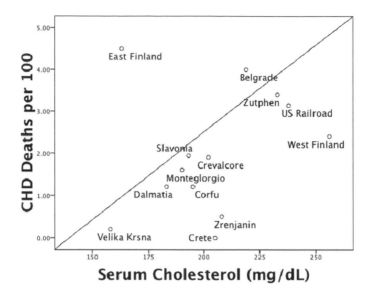

Serum Cholesterol (mg/dL)

Fig. 7.1 Relationship between median total cholesterol level in Seven countries and the number of people dying from coronary artery disease within 10 years following the cholesterol measurement at the country aggregate level, the correlation between cholesterol and death rate is 0.80. The equation suggests that for each 1-point increase in total cholesterol, the national death rate increases by 0.43. A 10-point increase in cholesterol would translate into an increase of 4.3 deaths per 1,000 persons in the population

The Framingham Heart Study, another well-known long-term research project, provided still stronger evidence of the relationship of high cholesterol rates and CVD. In this investigation, the residents of Framingham, MA, had their blood cholesterol measured and were followed over a course of many years. The study showed that those with high blood cholesterol were significantly more likely to have heart attacks and to die from heart disease than those with lower cholesterol levels. Cholesterol predicted CVD in every subgroup. For instance, high cholesterol was predictive of bad health outcomes for men and for women, for white and for nonwhite participants, for the well-educated and for the less-educated. It predicted heart attacks in people who were overweight or thin, and in both smokers and nonsmokers [2].

Progress in molecular biology has allowed scientists to breakdown the cholesterol into smaller constitute components. In recent years, subfractions or subdivisions of various cholesterol molecules have been identified. LDL cholesterol is considered the "bad" cholesterol—the one most likely responsible for the disease process that narrows the coronary arteries. High-density lipoprotein (HDL) cholesterol is considered the "good" cholesterol. These molecules are less numerous than LDL cholesterol but appear to have the opposite effect—they seem to reduce the tendency of arteries to narrow. It has been hypothesized that HDL carries cholesterol and fat away from the artery wall.

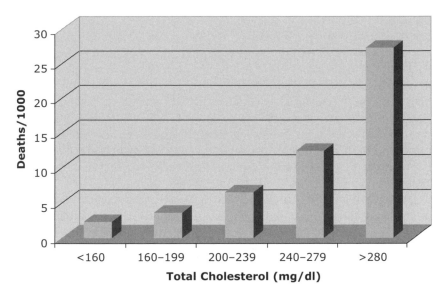

Fig. 7.2 CHD deaths by total cholesterol

Higher levels of HDL cholesterol might also be related to a slower build-up of plaque in the arteries and a reduced risk of CVD.

Figure 7.2 shows the relationship between total cholesterol levels and age-adjusted rates of heart disease. The data come from another well-known study, the Multiple Risk Factors Intervention Trial (MRFIT). This study involved 69,205 men aged 35–39 years who were observed and then followed over at least 16 years. The graph shows a very systematic relationship between total cholesterol and death from heart disease [3].

Epidemiologists, in their work analyzing the factors that influence the health of large populations, eventually focus on interventions. They are often not satisfied by merely showing the correlation between a risk factor and health outcomes. They want convincing evidence that a particular intervention will work and will improve the public health. In the case of cholesterol-lowering, this evidence has now accumulated. The National Heart, Lung, and Blood Institute conducted one landmark study through a national network of universities. The research group was known as the Lipid Research Clinics. The group conducted the Coronary Primary Prevention Trial (CPPT) that randomly assigned 3,806 men with high cholesterol but no symptoms of heart disease to either a cholesterol-lowering drug called cholestyrmanine or a placebo. The study was double-blinded. That means that neither the patients nor the experimenters knew whether a particular patient was taking the actual drug or the placebo. Both groups had dietary counseling and had their cholesterol measured over the next 7 years. In addition, the groups were followed for cardiovascular outcomes and for mortality. The study began in the mid-1970s, and the results were first reported in 1984.

The blood cholesterol was 8.5 percent lower in the group taking the drug in comparison with that in the placebo group. There was a 24-percent reduction in deaths from CVD. This led advocates of cholesterol-lowering to state that there was a 2-percent decrease in CVD for every 1-percent decrease in cholesterol. However, the absolute risk change was not remarkably strong. Among 1,900 participants taking the placebo, 38 individuals, or 2 percent, died of CVD. In comparison, 30 of the 1,906 subjects, 1.6 percent, in the cholestyrmanine group died of CVD. The absolute risk change was about 0.4 percent—four-tenths of 1 percentage point. These numbers focus only on deaths from CVD. Considering all causes of death, there was no difference between those taking cholestyrmanine and those using placebo [4, 5].

The results of the CPPT can be made to look as though cholestyrmanine is a great success or barely more than a flop, depending on how they are presented. Figure 7.3 shows a big difference in death rates between the medicated and the placebo groups. The presentation collapses the y-axis of the graph to 2 percentage points, thus dramatizing a difference in death rates that is only about 0.4 percent. In contrast, Fig. 7.4 offers a view of the same data but presented in such a way as to focus on the chances of *not* dying of heart disease over the 7 years. The y-axis is not collapsed. The chances of not dying of heart disease were very high for both groups—98.0 percent for the placebo group and 98.4 percent for the cholestyrmanine group. The advantage of taking the drug, as seen in this view of the data, is greatly diminished, almost to the point of disappearing.

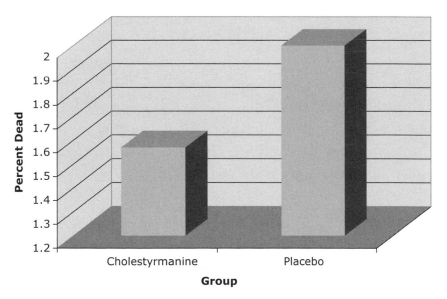

Fig. 7.3 Percentage of participants who had died of cardiovascular disease after 7 years of cholestyrmanine or placebo in the CPPT

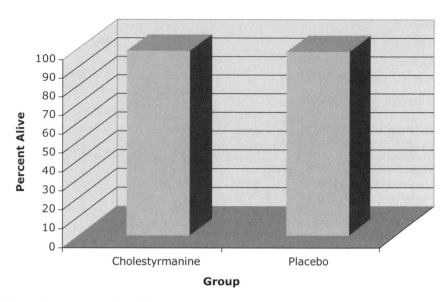

Fig. 7.4 Percentage of participants not dying of cardiovascular disease after 7 years of cholystramine or placebo in the CPPT

The CPPT was particularly important because it provided the scientific justification for the national campaign to lower cholesterol. Since the publication of the study in January 1984, several trials have evaluated newer cholesterol-lowering drugs known as statins. Perhaps the best example is the ASCAPS/TEXCAPS trial. In this study, those with elevated cholesterol were randomly assigned to take lovastatin (20–40 mg/day) or a placebo. Participants took the drug for nearly 5 years and were followed up for nearly 7 years. There was a 34-percent reduction in heart attacks and a 21-percent reduction in death from heart disease. However, there was no change in the number of people who had died when all causes of death were taken into consideration. Furthermore, the absolute risk reduction remained small. For example, 2.4 percent of the participants taking lovastatin had heart attacks while 3.6 percent of those taking the placebo had these events. The absolute risk change was about 1.2 percent. In terms of cardiovascular death, the difference was 0.5 percent for those taking lovastatin versus 0.6 percent for those taking placebo. In other words, there was a difference in CHD death rates of one person in every thousand.

The most challenging issue concerned the level at which screening for high cholesterol should begin. As noted above, there is relatively little controversy that people who are at high risk for heart attacks or death from heart disease should be treated. For these individuals, taking cholesterol-lowering medications is clearly worth the risk. But how about for people who are at the low end of the risk continuum? Over the last few decades, the National

Cholesterol Education Program has become increasingly aggressive in their recommendations.

Cholesterol Screening

Following the CPPT [4], the National Cholesterol Education Program argued for the aggressive management of elevated serum cholesterol. The arguments in favor of population-based cholesterol-lowering are multiple. Perhaps the two most persuasive arguments come from the MRFIT [3] and the British Medical Research Council/British Heart Foundation (BHF) Heart Protection Study [6]. The MRFIT study demonstrated that the relationship between total cholesterol and death from coronary heart disease was systematic and independent of the level of total cholesterol when participants entered the study. Reducing total cholesterol from 300 to 280, for example, provided the same percentage reduction in death from coronary disease as would be afforded someone reducing total cholesterol from 220 to 200 [3]. Ironically, the MRFIT study was an intervention trial which failed to demonstrate a benefit for intervening on risk factors [7]. Although the interventions failed to change the death rates, the researchers offered these conclusions based on observations of deaths among people who started the study with differing levels of cholesterol. The study did not show that interventions designed to reduce risk factors for heart disease resulted in actually reductions in risk.

Many difficulties in these analyses have now become apparent. First, the National Cholesterol Education Program recommended cholesterol-screening tests for all Americans independent of age, gender, or ethnicity. However, the published clinical trials at the time the policies were proposed were based exclusively on men, and there was no specific evidence for children [8]. A more recent meta-analysis of all of the published secondary prevention trials offers no evidence at all that cholesterol-lowering extends the life expectancy of women (see Table 7.1). Among nearly 2,400 women randomly assigned to take statins or placebos, there were 102 deaths among women taking the active drug and 103 deaths among women taking the placebo [9]. Although there were slightly more non-fatal heart attacks among women talking the cholesterol lowering drugs, they chances of dying of heart attacks were not affected.

A second concern was that the early clinical trials consistently failed to demonstrate improvements in life expectancy resulting from cholesterol-lowering [10]. In all early clinical trials, reductions in deaths from heart disease were offset by increases in deaths from other causes [11]. For example, the CPPT showed that a drug effectively lowered cholesterol in comparison with placebo. Furthermore, those taking the cholesterol-lowering medication were significantly less likely to die of heart disease than those taking the placebo. However, over the time period these participants were followed, there were more deaths from other causes among those taking the drug, and

Table 7.1 Summary of Meta-analysis summarizing the effects of cholesterol lowering for 11,435 women in six clinical trials (adapted from Walsh and Pegnone [9])

Number of women studied		Number of Deaths		Percent Death	
Non Fatal Heart Attack					
Placebo	Statin	Placebo	Statin	Placebo	Statin
1602	1588	93	66	5.50	4.16
Deaths from Heart Attack					
Placebo	Statin	Placebo	Statin	Placebo	Statin
1205	1188	103	102	8.54	8.58

the chances of being alive over the time span of the study were comparable in the two groups [5]. More recent evidence also demonstrates systematic increases in deaths from other causes for those taking cholesterol-lowering agents. Biological mechanisms for these increases have been proposed. Several studies document a relationship between low dietary fats and low cholesterol levels and a reduction in serotonin activity [12]. The early studies used resin drugs like cholestyrmanine that worked by binding bile acids and shutting down the natural production of cholesterol by the human body. The introduction of the statin medications largely silenced this controversy. Statins work through a different mechanism. Statins reduce cholesterol biosynthesis, mainly in the liver by modifying lipid metabolism. Studies involving statins tended to show reductions in both deaths from heart disease and from total mortality [13, 14]. Nevertheless, some controversy remained. The Medical Research Counsel (MRC) and BHF Heart Protection Study, published in 2002, was particularly important because it was large ($n = 20,536$) and randomized [6]. Perhaps the most interesting finding was that simvastatin, given to a wide range of individuals at risk for coronary disease, had broadly positive effects. There was a benefit in terms of CHD mortality irrespective of the initial cholesterol concentrations. Consumption of 40 mg of simvastatin daily was associated with reductions in MI, stroke, and the number of revascularization procedures (such as coronary bypass, angioplasty, and the insertion of stents). The study has been interpreted as suggesting the need for greater use of statin drugs in the population [6]. However, while the relative risk reduction afforded by the statins appears fairly constant over all risk groups, the absolute risk reduction is much smaller in those at lower risk. Those who are initially at high risk reduce their changes of dying significantly, while those whose cholesterol levels are relatively low reduce their personal risk only slightly. Furthermore, questions have been raised about the value of statins for low-risk women. The Walsh and Pignone meta-analysis (cited in Table 7.1) included six trials of lipid-lowering. The trials included 11,435 women without CVD. In these trials, women taking lipid-lowering drugs had about the same risk of dying of heart disease or of all causes as did women taking placebo [9]. For example, averaged across six studies 103 of 1,205 (8.54 percent) women taking placebo died in comparison with 102 of 1,188 (8.58 percent) taking statin drugs. Questions have also been raised about the rationale for statin therapy in older adults. For example, Packard and colleagues noted that LDL cholesterol is neither a good predictor of outcome nor a response to therapy in adults older than age 70. HDL cholesterol or the ratio of total to HDL may offer more information [15, 16]. While it is difficult to deny the value of statins for people truly at risk for early death due to high cholesterol, there may be a tendency to overprescribe the drugs to people who less clearly benefit from them. These include women, particularly those in the near normal ranges for cholesterol, the elderly, and both men and women with no other risk factors and whose cholesterol levels are near normal.

In any epidemiological study, only a small portion of the general population in each diagnostic category will be diagnosed. For example, it has been estimated 52 million Americans have serum cholesterol levels deserving attention, while the number in active treatment is a small fraction of potential cases [17]. Even among those who have an identified diagnosis, not all are assigned to treatment. And still furthermore, among those given treatment, between 15 and 90 percent do not adhere to physician recommendations. Concern that the public was not gaining the optimal benefit of treatment led to the development of treatment guidelines. Among many guidelines available, perhaps the most influential are the third revision of the Adult Treatment Protocol of the National Cholesterol Education Program.

Atp III

The third report of the National Cholesterol Education Program (NCEP) expert panel on detection, evaluation, and treatment of high cholesterol in adults, popularly called ATP III [18], is the current standard for cholesterol screening and treatment. ATP III is the third step in an evolutionary process. The first report (ATP I, published in 1988 outlined the strategy for the prevention of heart disease for adults with LDL >160 mg/dl and for those with high cholesterol (LDL 130–159 mg/dl). The second report (APT II, 1995) expanded APT I by discussing the intensive management of LDL cholesterol for people who had established heart disease. ATP III, published in 2001, called for more intensive intervention. Departing from previous recommendations, ATP III identified LDL cholesterol levels from 130 to 159 mg/dl as borderline high and total cholesterol levels between 200 and 239 mg/dl as borderline high for otherwise low-risk individuals. The report recommends lifestyle intervention for those with borderline high LDL or total cholesterol but also acknowledges that drug treatment may be appropriate for those who fail lifestyle interventions. Direct-to-consumer advertising sponsored by the pharmaceutical industry emphasizes that the majority of patients fail dietary interventions and that patients should speak to their doctors about drug therapy. (See, for example, www.Lipitor.com.)

The ATP III report discusses the cost-effectiveness of treatment, recognizing that drug therapy is expensive. However, it also dismisses some cost concerns by suggesting that drug prices are likely to decline in the future. ATP III also suggests that the threshold for considering treatment should be an LDL level of 130 mg/dl. Following the publication of the Heart Protection Study [19], the guidelines were revised to lower the threshold to 100 mg/dl [20] for people with other risk factors for heart disease.

Concerns and Conflicts of Interest

One concern is that most studies used to create guidelines are funded by the pharmaceutical industry. For example, one study found that 81 percent of clinical practice guidelines authors had interactions with the pharmaceutical industry, and 59 percent had relationships with companies whose drugs were evaluated in the guideline they authored [21]. The NCEP guidelines on cholesterol were based on several major studies (e.g., 4S, AFCAPS/TexCAPS, WOS) that were sponsored by the pharmaceutical industry. After the observation of the connection between industry and the development of national guidelines, disclosure requirements have become more stringent. Nevertheless, most of our current guidance were developed in an era when most guideline developers had strong financial ties to the pharmaceutical industry.

How Many People are Affected by the Changing Definitions?

Using data from the NHANES, we reevaluated the proportion of the adult population affected by the change in guidelines published in ATP III. The distribution of LDL cholesterol in the general US population, and for the US population age 60 or older, is shown in Fig. 7.5. The ATP III guidelines suggest that optimal levels of LDL cholesterol are below 70 mg/dl. However, that level is achieved by very few of us. Considering the entire adult population in the USA, only about 7 percent are at this level. Ninety-three percent of us have levels that are higher. For adults over age 60, 97 percent have LDL values higher than 70 mg/dl. The first threshold for clinical concern is 100 mg/dl. According to the analysis of the NHANES data, about 70 percent of the adult population of the USA falls into that category. In other words, the guidelines suggest that close to 70 percent of the population needs treatment or attention. According to our analysis of the NHANES data, 84 percent of adults over age 60 have LDL levels higher than 100, so 85 in each 100 might need attention for cholesterol management.

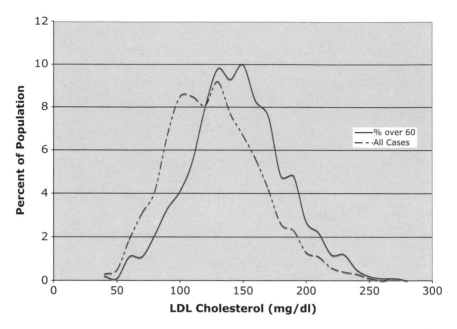

Fig. 7.5 Distribution of LDL cholesterol for all participants and those older than 60 years in NHANES III

The ATP III argues that there is a linear relationship between an individual's level of LDL cholesterol and the chances of heart attacks or deaths. The authors of the report even provided a nice-looking graph showing this relationship (see Fig. 7.6). The argument is that those who lower their LDL cholesterol from 170 to 160 gain about the same amount as those who lower their LDL cholesterol from 110 to 100. However, look at the graph more carefully. This figure was actually taken directly from the publication from the National Cholesterol Education Program. The *y*-axis on the graph is in logarithmic rather than

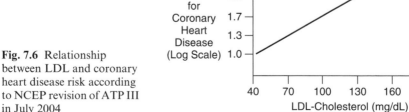

Fig. 7.6 Relationship between LDL and coronary heart disease risk according to NCEP revision of ATP III in July 2004

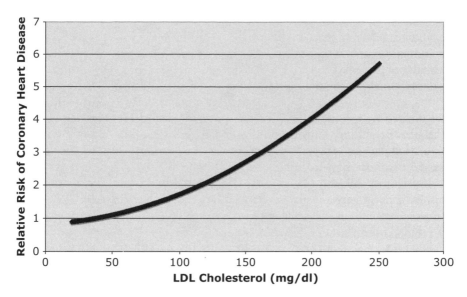

Fig. 7.7 Relationship between LDL and coronary heart disease risk using linear scale of risk

regular linear units. As with blood pressure, the relationship between risk factor and outcome is not linear. It is log-linear. Although the label in the figure clearly states that the *y*-axis data are on a log scale, the graph is deceptive because it appears to show a linear trend. There are no tick marks on the *y*-axis that would give the reader the impression that the scale is not in linear units. In addition, Fig. 7.6 disguises some of the relationship by excluding the small groups of the population with very low or very high LDL levels. Figure 7.7 redraws the relationship using natural units on the *y*-axis and the full range of LDL values (as reported in the NHANES survey) along the *x*-axis. Those who start with lower levels of LDL cholesterol gain significantly less than those who start with high levels of LDL cholesterol. This fits data from actual studies, such as the MRFIT (see Fig. 7.8).

Fig. 7.8 Six-year CHD mortality by total serum cholesterol for 356,222 men aged 35–57 years screened for the MRFIT study

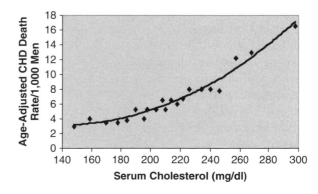

How Many Will Progress to CVD?

Pharmaceutical advertising suggests statin therapy for patients with mildly elevated LDL cholesterol and without other risk factors. However, statins have not been studied in populations without risk factors. Table 7.2 summarizes the entry criteria in several of the major recent clinical trials. These are the exact trials used as the rationale for the recent revision of ATP III. The first column lists the study and the middle column summarizes the population under study. The third column of the table which shows the entry criteria for the studies indicates that none of these trials used adults who did not have heart disease or did not have established risk factors. The benefits for lowering cholesterol in adults with relatively normal levels of LDL cholesterol are a bit less clear because these populations have not been studied in lipid-lowering trials.

In collaboration with UCSD medical student Doc Khagali, we recently evaluated the benefits of cholesterol lowering for hypothetical situations. We considered three hypothetical cases. The first was a 55-year-old nonsmoker with an HDL of 50 mg/dl and untreated systolic hypertension of 120 mmHg. The second case involved a higher risk patient, a 60-year-old nonsmoker with an HDL of 30 mg/dl and untreated systolic blood pressure of 140 mmHg. The third hypothetical case was the highest risk: a 65-year-old smoker with an HDL of 30 mg/dl and treated systolic blood pressure of 130 mmHg. Figure 7.9 shows the absolute risk reduction in women under these three hypothetical conditions. For those with initially low levels of total cholesterol, treatment provides almost

Table 7.2 Entry criteria in trials used as the basis for the ATP-III revised guidelines (from Kaplan and Ong, 2007 [22]) [11]

Study	Population	Entry criteria
Heart Protection Study [6]	20,536 adults, ages 40–80 in United Kingdom	Coronary disease, other occlusive artery disease, or diabetes
Prospective Study of Pravastatin in the Elderly at Risk (PROSPER) [23]	5,804 adults, ages, 70–82	History of heart disease or CVD risk factors
Antihypertensive and Lipid-Lowering Treatment to Prevent Heart Attack (ALLHAT) [24]	10,355 adults 55 years or older	LDL levels between 120 and 189 mg/dl and triglycerides <350 mg/dl
Anglo-Scandinavian Cardiac Outcomes Trial-Lipid Lowing Arm (ASCOT-LLA) [25]	19,342 patients ages 40–79 years	All had hypertension and at least 3 other CHD risk factors
Pravastatin or Atorvastatin Evaluation and Infection-Thrombolysis in Myocardial Infarction 22 (PROVE IT) [26]	4,162 patients from Australia, Canada, France, Germany, Italy, Spain, the United Kingdom, or the United States	All participants had been hospitalized for acute coronary syndrome within 10 days prior to randomization

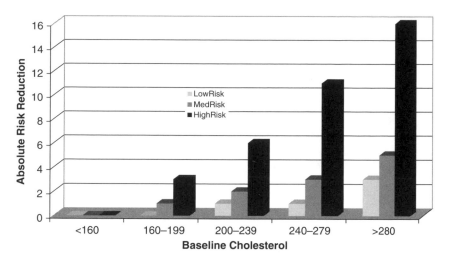

Fig. 7.9 Change in absolute risk reduction for three hypothetical cases. (From Khalegi and Kaplan, 2007 [27])

no benefit in any case. For those with higher levels of LDL cholesterol, treatment offers the most benefit for the high-risk patient. In this case, there may be an absolute risk reduction of about 16 percent. For the intermediate-risk patient, the absolute risk reduction is about 5 percent. And it is only about 3 percent for the low-risk patient. In other words, the three patients do not benefit equally from treatment. High-risk patients stand to gain significantly more than low-risk patients.

We can also consider the cost-effectiveness of those interventions. In this case, we considered the number of dollars required for 1 percentage point of absolute risk reduction. For the patient without other risk factors and a relatively normal level of total cholesterol, it would cost about $1,200 to reduce the chance of dying of heart disease by 1 percent. For the medium- and high-risk patient, the cost per percentage point of absolute risk reduction is about $400. For those who initially have high levels of total cholesterol and other risk factors, intervention may reduce the chances of dying by 1 percentage point for only about $50.

Finally, we estimated the expected benefit for someone lowering his or her cholesterol from 110 to 100. This can be calculated from ATP III Cholesterol Management Guidelines that are available on the National Cholesterol Education Program website. The site also includes a risk calculator.

Consider the hypothetical case of a 55-year-old male with a total cholesterol of 180 mg/dl, and LDL cholesterol of 110 mg/dl and an HDL cholesterol of 48 mg/dl. The person has no other risk factors. The 10-year mortality risk is less than 10 percent. That remains less than 10 percent when lowering cholesterol by 10 mg/dl. In fact, the percentage risk change is not distinguishable by the formula. The absolute risk change is near 0.

Conclusions

Elevated serum cholesterol is a risk factor for mortality from heart disease. Those with high levels of serum cholesterol should be treated. Treatment works, and it results in reductions in heart attacks and deaths from CVD.

However, energized by the value of cholesterol-lowering for people at risk for heart disease, advocates have become convinced that people with more normal cholesterol levels should also be treated. The National Cholesterol Education Program now promotes lower thresholds for the treatment of serum cholesterol. In fact, the newest guidelines identify nearly 90 percent of American adults as in need of monitoring or treatment. It has been suggested that those with initially lower levels of serum cholesterol may benefit just as much as those with higher levels. However, the data do not support this argument. The relationship between cholesterol and health outcomes is not linear. Instead, it is log-linear. In other words, those with initially low levels of LDL cholesterol do not reduce their risks to the extent that those with high initial levels of high LDL cholesterol reduce risk. Furthermore, those with initially low risks of LDL cholesterol are significantly less likely to die of heart disease. Taking medication is not completely without risk. These individuals may be exposed to side effects of medication without clear evidence that they obtain the benefits.

The American Heart Association, in collaboration with the pharmaceutical industry and the NIH, has promoted the "Know your Number" campaign. The purpose is to get people to know their cholesterol values. At least from the perspective of the pharmaceutical industry, the benefits of this campaign are quite clear. Even using previous definitions of high cholesterol, more than half of the adult population was eligible for diagnosis. With the new definitions, the proportion of the population eligible for treatment approaches 70 percent. For older adults, it approaches 100 percent. The more people know their number, the more people are likely to get prescriptions for products manufactured by these companies. Drugs used to treat high cholesterol are not like drugs used to treat other illnesses. In contrast to an antibiotic, which is used for a brief period in order to eliminate a bacterial disease, cholesterol-lowering drugs are used for a lifetime. The stakes are enormous. In Chapter 9, we will consider other consequences in promoting drugs to manage common illnesses.

References

1. Keys AB. *Coronary heart disease in seven countries.* New York: American Heart Association; 1970.
2. Wilson PW, D'Agostino RB, Levy D, Belanger AM, Silbershatz H, Kannel WB. Prediction of coronary heart disease using risk factor categories. *Circulation.* May 12 1998;97(18):1837–1847.
3. Stamler J, Daviglus ML, Garside DB, Dyer AR, Greenland P, Neaton JD. Relationship of baseline serum cholesterol levels in 3 large cohorts of younger men to long-term coronary,

cardiovascular, and all-cause mortality and to longevity. *JAMA*. Jul 19 2000;284(3):311–318.

4. The Lipid Research Clinics Coronary Primary Prevention Trial results. II. The relationship of reduction in incidence of coronary heart disease to cholesterol lowering. *JAMA*. Jan 20 1984;251(3):365–374.

5. The Lipid Research Clinics Coronary Primary Prevention Trial results. I. Reduction in incidence of coronary heart disease. *JAMA*. Jan 20 1984;251(3):351–364.

6. MRC/BHF Heart Protection Study of cholesterol lowering with simvastatin in 20,536 high-risk individuals: a randomised placebo-controlled trial. *Lancet*. Jul 6 2002;360(9326):7–22.

7. Multiple risk factor intervention trial: risk factor changes and mortality results. Multiple Risk Factor Intervention Trial Research Group. *JAMA*. Sep 24 1982;248(12):1465–1477.

8. Kaplan RM. Two pathways to prevention. *Am Psychol*. 2000;55(4):382–396.

9. Walsh JM, Pignone M. Drug treatment of hyperlipidemia in women. *JAMA*. May 12 2004;291(18):2243–2252.

10. Kaplan RM. Behavioral epidemiology, health promotion, and health services. *Med Care*. May 1985;23(5):564–583.

11. Muldoon MF, Manuck SB, Matthews KA. Lowering cholesterol concentrations and mortality: a quantitative review of primary prevention trials. *Brit Phycol J*. Aug 11 1990;301(6747):309–314.

12. Golomb BA. Cholesterol and violence: is there a connection? *Ann Intern Med*. 1998;128(6):478–487.

13. Caro J, Klittich W, McGuire A, et al. The West of Scotland coronary prevention study: economic benefit analysis of primary prevention with pravastatin [see comments]. *Brit Phycol J (Clinical Research Ed.)*. 1997;315(7122):1577–1582.

14. Downs JR, Clearfield M, Weis S, et al. Primary prevention of acute coronary events with lovastatin in men and women with average cholesterol levels: results of AFCAPS/TexCAPS. Air Force/Texas Coronary Atherosclerosis Prevention Study. *JAMA*. 1998;279(20):1615–1622.

15. Packard CJ, Ford I, Robertson M, et al. Plasma lipoproteins and apolipoproteins as predictors of cardiovascular risk and treatment benefit in the PROspective Study of Pravastatin in the Elderly at Risk (PROSPER). *Circulation*. Nov 15 2005;112(20):3058–3065.

16. Criqui MH, Golomb BA. Low and lowered cholesterol and total mortality. *J Am Coll Cardiol*. Sep 1 2004;44(5):1009–1010.

17. Sempos CT, Cleeman JI, Carroll MD, et al. Prevalence of high blood cholesterol among US adults: an update based on guidelines from the second report of the National Cholesterol Education Program Adult Treatment Panel. *JAMA*. 1993;269(23):3009–3014.

18. Executive Summary of the Third Report of the National Cholesterol Education Program (NCEP) Expert Panel on Detection, Evaluation, And Treatment of High Blood Cholesterol In Adults (Adult Treatment Panel III). *JAMA*. May 16 2001;285(19):2486–2497.

19. Collins R, Armitage J, Parish S, Sleigh P, Peto R. MRC/BHF Heart Protection Study of cholesterol-lowering with simvastatin in 5963 people with diabetes: a randomised placebo-controlled trial. *Lancet*. Jun 14 2003;361(9374):2005–2016.

20. Gurm HS, Hoogwerf B. The Heart Protection Study: high-risk patients benefit from statins, regardless of LDL-C level. *Cleve Clin J Med*. Nov 2003;70(11):991–997.

21. Choudhry NK, Stelfox HT, Detsky AS. Relationships between authors of clinical practice guidelines and the pharmaceutical industry. *JAMA*. 2002;287(5):612–617.

22. Kaplan RM, Ong M. Rationale and Public Health Implications of Changing CHD Risk Factor Definitions. *Annu Rev Public Health*. 2007;28:312–344.

23. Shepherd J, Blauw GJ, Murphy MB, et al. Pravastatin in elderly individuals at risk of vascular disease (PROSPER): a randomised controlled trial. *Lancet*. Nov 23 2002;360(9346):1623–1630.

24. Major outcomes in moderately hypercholesterolemic, hypertensive patients randomized to pravastatin vs usual care: the Antihypertensive and Lipid-Lowering Treatment to Prevent Heart Attack Trial (ALLHAT-LLT). *JAMA*. Dec 18 2002;288(23):2998–3007.
25. Sever PS, Dahlof B, Poulter NR, et al. Prevention of coronary and stroke events with atorvastatin in hypertensive patients who have average or lower-than-average cholesterol concentrations, in the Anglo-Scandinavian Cardiac Outcomes Trial – Lipid Lowering Arm (ASCOT-LLA): a multicentre randomised controlled trial. *Lancet*. Apr 5 2003;361(9364):1149–1158.
26. Cannon CP, McCabe CH, Belder R, Breen J, Braunwald E. Design of the Pravastatin or Atorvastatin Evaluation and Infection Therapy (PROVE IT)-TIMI 22 trial. *Am J Cardiol*. Apr 1 2002;89(7):860–861.
27. Khaleghi M, Kaplan RM. Effects of Changing Illness Thresholds on Healthcare Costs and Health Outcomes. Unpublished paper, University of California, San Diego, 2007.

Chapter 8
Diabetes, Obesity, and the Metabolic Syndrome

Diabetes mellitus (DM) or diabetes, as we usually call it, is a major medical, personal, and public-health problem. Diabetes is a chronic disease associated with abnormally high levels of glucose (sugars) in the blood. A rise in glucose occurs when foods are consumed. Glucose from blood is an energy source for cells and tissues throughout the body. However, utilization of glucose requires a hormone, insulin, that allows the glucose to be used. Diabetes occurs when the body does not make enough insulin or when cells cannot adequately make use of the available insulin. In 2006, the American Diabetes Association (ADA) estimated that 20.8 million people, roughly 7 percent of the US population, had diabetes. Among these, 14.6 million have been diagnosed, and 6.2 million are unaware they have the condition. Another 41 million have "pre-diabetes,"[1] a condition many experts believe leads to diabetes.

The incidence of the disease in the US population varies with age. For those over 60, more than 20 percent have the disease. Each year approximately 1.5 million new cases of diabetes are diagnosed, or over 4,000 each day. Diabetes is the sixth leading cause of death in the USA. Each year approximately 200,000 deaths are directly or indirectly attributable to the disease, while many other deaths are associated with the complications of diabetes [2]. There are at least two types of diabetes. Type 1 requires use of insulin for survival and is the most severe form of the disease. Only about 10 percent of people with diabetes are dependent on insulin. The others have type 2 diabetes, a form not requiring insulin injections for most people. The most important risk factor of type 2 diabetes is being overweight or obese. The proportion of the population with diabetes increases with age because most new cases are type 2.

The prevalence of the disease also seems to vary from one racial or ethnic group to another. Native Americans, African-Americans, Hispanics, and Pacific Islanders, for example, may be at increased risk for the disease (see Fig. 8.1).

It is interesting to look back at ADA reports over the last few years. For example, according to the organization's 2000 data, there were only about half as many cases of diabetes as there are today. Does this really mean we are experiencing a snowballing epidemic? Despite the increased number of cases, the number of deaths from diabetes has not changed much over these last few years. We will explore this problem in more detail, but first, we will consider the basic pathophysiology of diabetes.

R.M. Kaplan, *Disease, Diagnoses, and Dollars*, DOI 10.1007/978-0-387-74045-4_8,
© Springer Science+Business Media, LLC 2009

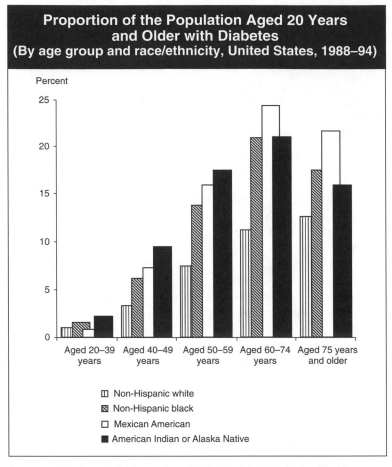

Sources: Harris et al. *Diabetes Care* 21(4):518–24, 1998; Indian Health
Service national outpatient database.

Fig. 8.1 Proportion of the population age 20 years and older with diabetes by age groups and
race/ethnicity

Pathophysiology

Many different factors may cause the onset of diabetes, and its course and
prognosis vary among individuals. The technical medical term *diabetes mellitus*
actually covers several separate and distinct conditions. The term DM is used to
separate the common condition from other rare diabetic diseases such as a
kidney disease known as *diabetes insipidus* and a specialized form of diabetes
that occurs during pregnancy known as *gestational diabetes*. The two most
common forms of DM are type 1, or insulin-dependent DM (IDDM), and

type 2, non-IDDM (NIDDM). Type 1 is considered to be the most severe form, and individuals in this subclass require insulin injections to preserve life. There appears to be no epidemic of type 1 diabetes. The rates in the population have been relatively steady for the last few decades.

Those with type 2 DM may use insulin to correct high blood glucose levels but do not require an external source of insulin in order to survive. Type 2 diabetes is by far the most common type of diabetes, although we typically think of a diabetic patient as one who requires insulin. Type 1 diabetes is a relatively rare form of the condition, accounting for less than 10 percent of all cases, while type 2 accounts for about 90 percent. Among these with type 2, 60–90 percent are overweight [3], and some evidence suggests that weight loss can be of substantial benefit to these individuals [4]. Thus, the ADA now recommends diet and exercise as the primary interventions for control of type 2 diabetes [1]. In other words, they recommend that patients be given a serious trial of behavioral intervention before being exposed to drug treatment. Nevertheless, an increasing number of people are being given medications for diabetes.

Type 1 and type 2 diabetes are very different diseases. In each case, environmental factors acting in concert with genetic susceptibility may be important precursors. There is substantial evidence that type 1 diabetes has a genetic component. People with certain genetic markers for human leukocyte antigens (HLAs) are at increased risk for developing type 1 diabetes. Siblings of children with type 1 diabetes are at increased risk of developing the condition; in fact, their chances are seven times the rate in the general population [5]. However, if the condition were purely genetic, we would expect perfect concordance, or correspondence, in identical twins, and this is not the case: Only between 20 and 50 percent of the identical twins of those with type 1 diabetes actually develop the disease.

The glucose system is *homeostatic,* meaning it is self-balancing. The body attempts to maintain blood glucose at a relatively constant level. If a person does not eat food, insulin secretions stimulate release of stored glucose from the liver. The normally functioning person makes a series of internal adjustments that result in relatively steady levels of blood glucose throughout the day. In the absence of appropriate insulin levels, or when insulin receptors are defective, blood sugar levels rise. At the same time, hungry cells starve and begin to burn other fuels as an energy source. When cells burn fat as an energy source, they release ketones as a metabolic by-product. These ketones can be released into the blood and can cause the blood to become acidic. Severe cases of this problem are known as *ketoacidosis* (implying that the blood has become acidic from ketones). Severe ketoacidosis can result in coma and death. The kidneys separate elements that are retained in the blood supply and waste products that are eliminated in urine. When the blood sugar gets to a very high level, it may reach a point where the kidneys can no longer process it. As a result, some of the sugar "spills" into the urine. Thus, elevated levels of sugar in urine are sometimes an indicator of diabetes.

For those with type 2 diabetes, the picture is the opposite. Several decades ago, a test was developed to measure how much insulin the body produced. Until this time, it was believed that those with type 2 diabetes had difficulty producing insulin, as did those with insulin-dependent diabetes (type 1). However, the new tests demonstrated that subjects with type 2 diabetes actually had *higher* levels of insulin in response to sugar ingestion than did control subjects who did not have diabetes. This condition is known as hyperinsulinemia because it is associated with the overproduction (hyper) of insulin (insulinemia). A variety of researchers have demonstrated that hyperinsulinemia may be associated with obesity; in fact, the amount of excess body weight is related to the degree of hyperinsulinemia [6]. In other words, evidence suggests that type 2 diabetes might be associated not with too little but with too *much* insulin. Some of the more recent studies also suggest that type 2 diabetes is associated with insulin resistance, which results when the cells that normally process insulin do not function properly [7].

The reasons for insulin resistance are not known. However, it has been suggested that insulin resistance is an adaptive response to hyperinsulinemia. Some of the newer studies also suggest that type 2 diabetes is heterogeneous, meaning that different people have the condition for different reasons. Some people may overproduce insulin, some may produce about average amounts, and some may actually under-produce it. Some people may have problems with insulin receptors, while others may not [8].

It may be inappropriate to think of diabetes as a disease. Rather, it is an abnormality in metabolic control. However, poor metabolic control over a long period of time has serious health consequences because it is associated with breakdowns in nearly every system within the body. Some of the major complications of diabetes and poor metabolic control are heart disease, nephropathy, blindness, amputations of the feet and toes, and perinatal mortality and morbidity [1]. These are only a few of the many serious complications of the diabetes. So, control of diabetes is an important health goal.

The Changing Definition of Diabetes and Impaired Fasting Glucose

Both major types of diabetes are increasing, but not at the same rate, and not with the same path to serious consequences. Both forms of the disease are serious, but they behave differently, and that means individuals with the conditions tend to behave differently.

Type 1 diabetes has a high chance of causing sudden and dramatic complications that can quickly put a person in a life-threatening situation. Without immediate treatment, death is likely. Type 2 diabetes is also a serious disease, but many people have the condition without knowing it, since there can be relatively minor forms of the disease, and even in its most serious form, the progress of the disease may be hidden. The fears about diabetic complications among those with type 2 are, as a rule, less urgent and less alarming, but that only makes the condition harder to deal with.

The healthy human body does a good job of maintaining homeostasis in blood sugar. When we eat, our blood sugar goes up. In response, insulin is released to metabolize the glucose. Blood glucose is measured in blood plasma and is expressed as the number of milligrams for each deciliter of the measured plasma. This is expressed as mg/dl. Ordinarily, blood glucose is maintained between 80 and 120 mg/dl of blood. There are two common tests for or diabetes or pre-diabetes. The tests are called the fasting plasma glucose (FPG) test and the oral glucose tolerance test (OGTT). In FPG, if a person has a level of 126 mg/dl after having fasted for eight or more hours, it is presumed he or she has diabetes. OGTT requires a sample of blood to test glucose levels after a fast and then 2 hours after drinking a glucose-rich beverage. If the blood glucose level is at 200 mg/dl or higher 2 hours after consumption of the glucose-loaded drink, the person is assumed to have diabetes.

As for blood pressure (see Chapter 6) and cholesterol (Chapter 7), there have also been recent changes in the definition of DM and impaired fasting glucose (IFG), or pre-diabetes. Several years ago, the Expert Committee on the Diagnosis and Classification of Diabetes Mellitus recommended that the threshold for diabetes be changed from a fasting blood glucose level of 140–126 mg/dl [9]. With a simple change in disease definition, the prevalence of diabetes increased to 14 percent.

More recently, the Expert Committee on the Diagnosis and Classification of Diabetes Mellitus also proposed a new, lower limit for IFG [10], recommending that the lower limit for IFG should be reduced from 110 to 100 mg/dl. The rationale for their recommendation was the belief that metabolic and clinical complications of hyperglycemia rise sharply for those above the 100-mg/dl level. However, the committee noted that there was very little evidence that cardiovascular risk factors and all-causes mortality rates increase with IFG. They also noted that some studies did not support lowering the threshold [11, 12]. As part of their discussion, the group noted that lowering the threshold to 100 mg/dl would significantly increase the number of patients with a diagnostic label. The committee felt this was desirable because it would bring medical attention to more individuals. The committee argued that population studies from Mauritius [13] and from the Pima Indians from Arizona [14] supported the lower threshold. The only American population considered was the San Antonio Heart Study population, which has a high number of people who have some of Native American heritage [15].

IFG and Its Consequences

The ADA suggests that IFG, or pre-diabetes, is the pathway to full diabetes. Consequently, they urge the general population to be tested because elevated blood glucose may result in diabetic complications. But what do we really know about the long-term consequences of minor elevations in blood glucose? With colleagues at the University of California, San Diego, we evaluated the benefit of the new definition of IFG. In 1972–1974, 82 percent of an upper middle-class white community in California (Rancho Bernardo) was screened for heart disease risk factors as part of the Lipid Research Clinic Prevalence Program. The average age at baseline was 49.9 years. A follow-up visit was conducted from 1992 to 1996 and included approximately 75 percent of the surviving Rancho Bernardo cohort ($n = 1,781$). The study examined data from all the subjects who had valid plasma glucose values for both visits ($n = 1,494$).

Fasting plasma glucose levels were measured at both follow-up visits, and four categories of fasting plasma glucose were created: nonimpaired (less than 100 mg/dl), low IFG (100–110 mg/dl), IFG (111–126 mg/dl), and DM (greater than 126 mg/dl and/or diagnosed or taking diabetic medications). Each participant was placed in one of the four categories at the baseline (1972–1974) and were followed up 20 years later, during the first 1992–1996 follow-up visits. Diabetic complications were also measured at the second follow-up visits. These included kidney function and eye problems. A self-report questionnaire was used to ask questions relating to neuropathy, including three categories: (1) numbness or tingling, (2) loss of sensation in both hands or feet, and (3) decreased ability to feel temperature by touching. For this analysis, participants were scored as having neuropathy if they reported any one of the three symptoms. The questionnaire was also used to determine self-reported use of prescription medications for diabetes and whether a health professional had told the respondent that he or she had diabetes.

Among the 605 with FPG values less than 100 mg/dl at baseline, 502 (82.9 percent) maintained FPG values less than 100 mg/dl over the next 20 years. Only 14 of 605 (2.3 percent) with FPG values less than 100 mg/dl progressed to diabetes. For those 390 participants with baseline FPG values between 100 and 110, only 16 (4.1 percent) worsened to diabetes, while 7 percent of the 285 subjects with FPG values between 111 and 126 worsened to diabetes over the next 20 years. Those in the low-IFG category (FPG from 100 to 110 mg/dl) were not significantly more likely to develop diabetes than those with FPG values less than 100 mg/dl. However, there was a significant increase in chances of conversion to diabetes for those in 111–126 range in comparison to the nonimpaired but not the low-IFG groups. This effect was significant for men but not for women.

Table 8.1 summarizes three diabetic complications at follow-up by FPG levels at baseline. Those with initial FPG levels greater than 126 mg/dl at in the early 1970 s had a significantly higher probability of elevated urinary albumin/ creatinine ratios in the 1990 s compared with the nonimpaired group. However, those in the two categories of IFG were not significantly more likely to develop kidney complications 20 years later than those with FPG <100 mg/dl [16]. Several other studies are consistent with this analysis. A 6.8-year follow-up of 2,763 women with established heart disease did not find a relationship between the new definition of IFG (100–110 mg/dl) and the incident events of CHD, stroke, TIA, or CHF [17].

Table 8.1 Percentage of participants with complications in kidney (high albumin in urine), eye (retinopathy), and nerves (neuropathy), at 20 years after baseline breaking down by category of initial fasting plasma glucose: Rancho Bernardo, CA

FPG category in 1972–1974	Kidney $n = 171$	Eye $n = 32$	Nerve $n = 185$
<100	10.6	3.8	10.8
100–110	13.6	3.5	12.7
111–126	12.7	3.4	14.5
>126	19.5*	8.2	24.2**

FPG category >126 also includes medications for diabetes and doctor's diagnosis
*differs significantly from <100 group
** differs significantly from all comparison FPG groups

The cut point for a diagnosis is the threshold, above which people are considered to have a problem. In deciding on cut points, the committee also considered the cost. They stated, "We do not yet know the total benefit or the total cost to an individual who is designated at risk for diabetes by either test, by any criterion. The higher the ratio of benefit to cost, the lower the optimum cut point that should be selected." The committee felt that there was a cost advantage to lowering the threshold because complications of diabetes might be prevented. They cited the diabetes prevention program (DPP) as evidence [4]. On the other hand, lowering the threshold will mean that many people will be subjected to treatment even though they have a very low probability of complications. Furthermore, the DPP did not study isolated IFG; participants had to have IFG *and* impaired glucose tolerance.

Multiple studies have shown that lifestyle modifications or pharmacotherapy can delay or prevent the progression from impaired glucose control (as measured either by impaired glucose tolerance or IFG) [4, 18–21]. Only one study, the DPP [4], has compared lifestyle modifications and pharmacotherapy together.

The DPP study enrolled individuals with a fasting plasma glucose of 95–125 mg/dl and an OGTT of 140–199 mg/dl, which was considered elevated but not meeting the threshold for diabetes by the 1997 ADA guidelines. The DPP study had three arms that enrolled about 1,000 patients each—placebo, lifestyle intervention, and pharmacotherapy intervention (metformin), where the lifestyle intervention combined a healthy low-calorie, low-fat diet with a physical activity regimen of moderate intensity, such as brisk walking, for at least 150 minutes per week. The placebo rate of progression to diabetes in the DPP study was 11 per 100 person-years, and both the lifestyle intervention (by 58 percent) and the pharmacotherapy intervention (by 31 percent) reduced progression to diabetes, as compared with the placebo arm.

The DPP also included a cost/utility analysis. Quality of life was measured using the Quality of Well-Being Scale (QWB) [22]. The measure was chosen because it can be used to estimate Quality-adjusted life years (QALYs) [23]. These are years of life, with an adjustment for quality of life. The concept is discussed in more detail in Chapter 9. Over the course of 3 years, those randomly assigned to the lifestyle intervention accrued 0.050 more QALYs than those assigned a regular dose of metformin. Among the three interventions, the lifestyle approach was the most expensive (total cost US $27,065 in 2000). Metformin was less expensive ($25,937), while placebo was the least expensive option ($23,525). Although both interventions offer significant benefits over placebo or doing nothing, the cost/QALY for the lifestyle invention was significantly lower than for metformin. In other words, even though the lifestyle intervention was more expensive, it offers significantly better value for money.

So, there seems to be little evidence that fasting plasma glucose levels between 100 and 110 mg/dl are strong predictors of transition to diabetes, or the development of diabetic complications. These data stand in contrast to the recommendation of the Expert Committee on the Diagnosis and Classification of Diabetes Mellitus, which promoted lowering the threshold for IFG down to 100 mg/dl. My colleagues (Deborah Morton, Deborah Wingard, Elizabeth Barrett-Connor) and I believe that the selection of disease thresholds requires continuing thought and evaluation.

Obesity and Overweight

Obesity is a major public-health problem. In the early 1990 s, it was estimated that more than 300,000 adults in the USA died each year of causes related to obesity (Manson et al., 1991). According to the Centers for Disease Control and Prevention, no state at that time had an obesity rate of greater than 20 percent, but by 2001, just 10 years later, 29 states had obesity rates of 20 percent or more. The numbers were the cause for alarm. That the prevalence of obesity in the USA had increased 74 percent in the 1991–2001 decade suggested nothing less than an epidemic. Obesity not only increases the risk of mortality, but also is associated with losses in quality of life [24]. It has been suggested that obesity and overweight related problems are responsible for over 9 percent of the US Healthcare expenditures or over $92 billion in 2002 [25, 26].

Those who are obese, and those who fall into the less severe but still serious category of being overweight, live with not only increased risk of mortality, but a greater likelihood of losses in quality of life [24]. It has been suggested that obesity- and overweight-related problems are responsible for over 9 percent of the US healthcare expenditures, or over $92 billion in 2002 [25, 26].

Obesity is defined using a BMI. The BMI is calculated as an individual's weight in kilograms divided by the square of the height in meters, or kg/m^2. Those with a BMI of greater than 30 kg/m^2 are designated as obese. Those with a BMI of greater than 25 kg/m^2 are designated as overweight. Several years ago, the World Health Organization reduced its diagnosis threshold for overweight from a BMI of 27 to 25 kg/m^2.

The rationale for the threshold change was that BMI was systematically related to risk factors for heart disease. This is best represented in Fig. 8.2. A variety of studies show that BMI is related to blood pressure. For populations of both men

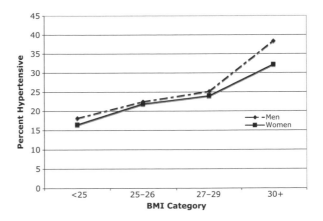

Fig. 8.2 Relationship between BMI category and the percentage of the male and female population with hypertension. Data from National Heart, Lung, and Blood Institute- public domain

and women, there is a positive correlation between rates of elevated BMI and rates of elevated blood pressure. The data in Fig. 8.2 come from the National Heart, Lung, and Blood Institute, Joint National Commission on High Blood Pressure and have been reported in documents from the National Heart, Lung and Blood Institute. For both men and women, there is a systematic relationship between increases in BMI and the percentage of people with hypertension.

The change in the definition of "overweight" had a substantial impact on the number of people in the population identified as being with the condition. Figure 8.3 shows the distribution of BMI based on the NHANES. This analysis considers people aged 40 years and older. In this group 49 percent of the population have a BMI greater than 25, 33 percent have a BMI greater than 27 or higher and about 20 percent have BMI a greater than 30. Changing the definition of overweight from a BMI of 27 kg/m^2 to a BMI of 25 kg/m^2 increased the number of proportion of people considered overweight or obese from about one-third to about one-half. In raw numbers, overweight of obese people increased from about 70 million to about 100 million.

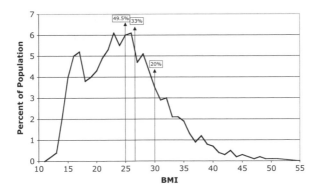

Fig. 8.3 Increase in the number of people identified as overweight when threshold was reduced from a BMI of 27–25. 49 percent of the population age 40 or over has a BMI greater than 25, 33 percent have BMI greater than 27, and about 20 percent have BMI greater than 30

One of the complicating factors is that individuals with substantial muscle mass have higher BMI scores. Consider elite athletes. Barry Bonds, the super-star baseball player, is 6 feet 2 inches tall and weighs 235 lbs. His BMI is 30.02. According to the definitions currently in use, Mr. Bonds is not just overweight, he is obese (see Fig. 8.4 to judge for yourself). Now, consider the author (shown in Fig. 8.4). I am 5 feet 9 inches tall and weigh just over 160 lbs. Although people rarely consider me to be overweight, my BMI is over 24. In other words, I am bordering on being overweight. In fact, nearly all American adults are over-weight by current standards. Figure 8.5 shows the trends in overweight accord-ing to the National Health and Nutritional Examination survey. As the figure clearly illustrates, there have been steady increases in the proportion of the population defined as overweight (left-hand portion of the figure) and obese (right-hand portion of the figure). In fact, it is now more difficult, according to the chart's data covering the period 1999–2002, to find either men or women who are *not* overweight (for more detailed information, see www.cdc.gov/nccdphp/dnpa/obesity/).

As noted above, being overweight is related to risk factors for heart disease. However, we must ask whether being overweight is really a risk factor for early

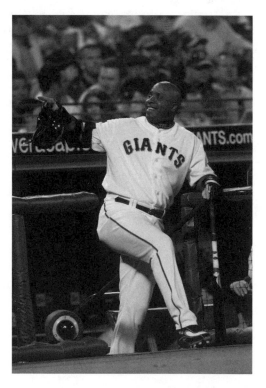

Fig. 8.4 (**a** and **b**) Barry Bonds is obese (BMI 30.2) while the author is on the boarder line of being overweight. You can judge for yourself (Courtesy of Justin Sullivan, Getty Images Sport)

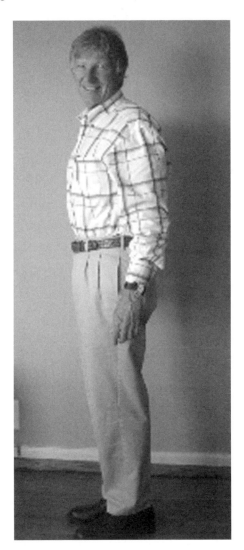

Fig. 8.4 (continued)

death or for loss in quality of life. In order to investigate this question, we aggregated data across major epidemiologic studies. These studies were well summarized by Allison and colleagues [27]. The results are presented in Fig. 8.6. Each line on the graph represents one of these major studies. The x-axis on the graph shows BMI and the y-axis shows the probability of all-causes mortality in these major studies. As the figure shows, the relationship is fairly flat in the range of BMIs from 25 to about 28 kg/m^2. Above the BMI of 28, there is a gradual increase in mortality. It has been argued that the relationship between

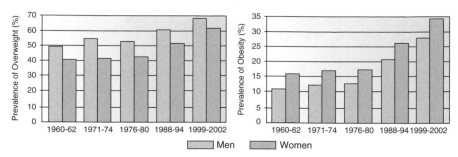

Time trends of age-adjusted prevalence of Overweight (BMI³ 25kg/m²) and obesity (BMI³ 30kg/m²)
in United States men and women who are 20 years of age and older.

Fig. 8.5 Time trends in the prevalence of overweight (BMI >25 *left side* of figure) and obese
(BMI >30) for men and women in the USA

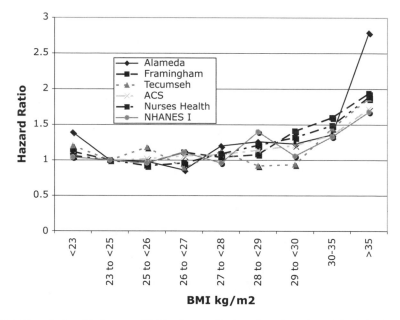

Fig. 8.6 The relationship between BMI and mortality based on six major epidemiologic studies
reviewed by Allison et al. [27]. Alameda = Alameda County Health Study, Framingham =$-
Framingham Heart Study, Tecumseh = Tecumseh Community Health Study, ACS = American
Cancer Society Cancer Prevention Study, Nurses Health = Nurses Health Study, NHANES-I
$-National Health and Nutrition Survey I Epidemiologic Follow-up Study. Hazard ratio is
defined as the ratio of mortality in relation of "normal" BMI of 23 to <25.

body weight and mortality is different for smokers and nonsmokers. However,
a separate examination of nonsmokers in these studies also showed that the
relationship between BMI and mortality is very flat between BMIs of 25 and
27 kg/m². On the basis of mortality risk, then, there appears to be no justification for changing the threshold for the definition of being overweight.

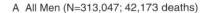

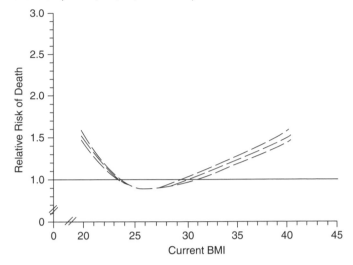

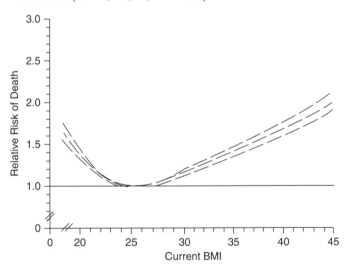

Fig. 8.7 The risk of death between 1995 and 2005 for AARP members by BMI. 1.0 defines the risk for those who are normal weight and the numbers on the y-axis define the risk in relation to these normal weight people. A value of 2.0, for example, suggests that people in this range are at twice the risk level as those who are normal weight. (From Adams et al. [28], Figs. 1 and 2.)

Another recent study of BMI and its relation to mortality was reported by Kenneth Adams and his colleagues in the August 24, 2006 issue of *The New England Journal of Medicine* [28]. The researchers studied 527,265 men and women who participated in an NIH study of AARP members. The participants self-reported their height and weight in 1995–1996 and were followed for mortality through 2005. During that interval, 42,173 men and 19,144 women died. Adams and associates concluded that excess weight was associated with an increasing risk of death. Yet, their data do not support the risk of BMIs in the 25–27 range. Figure 8.7 shows the curves Adams et al. fit for the relationship between BMI and death for both women and men. The relative risks of death are shown as the solid line, and the two dashed lines represent 95 percent confidence intervals. 1.0 defines the risk for those who are normal weight and the numbers on the y-axis define the risk in relation to these normal weight people. A value of 2.0, for example, suggests that people in this range are at twice the risk level as those who are normal weight. For both sexes, those in the 25–27 BMI range are at the lowest risk for death. For men, being in this range actually appears to be protective.

If body mass in the range of 25–27 kg/m^2 is not related to early death, is it related to quality of life? In order to investigate this question, we studied quality of life in the community of Rancho Bernardo, CA. A total of 1,326 adults with an average age of 72 years completed the Quality of Well-Being Scale (QWB), which is a general measure of health-related quality of life that places wellness on a continuum between death (scored as 0.0) to optimum health (scored as 1.0). These adults were also measured and weighed. The results of the analysis are presented in Fig. 8.8. The average BMI for all participants was 25.4, which is above the threshold for being overweight. The average quality of life score for people who were overweight but not obese was 0.695. This value was not

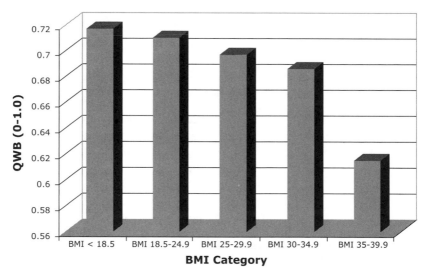

Fig. 8.8 Scores on a general quality of life measure—the quality of well-being scale (QWB) in relation to BMI category. (Data from the Rancho Bernardo Study)

Fig. 8.9 Man with
metabolic syndrome
(Courtesy of Gusto/Photo
Researchers, Inc.)

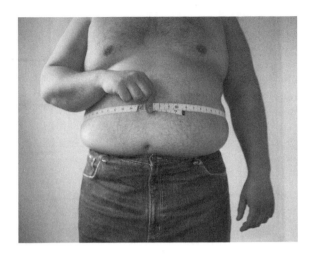

significantly different from the normal weight group's QWB rating of 0.709. Although there are slight decreases in quality of life with increasing BMI, it is only when people are very overweight (BMI greater than 35) that there are large and statistically significant changes in quality of life [24].

What does all this mean? Clearly, obesity is a major public-health problem. In fact, it is considered to be one of the most challenging problems we will face in the twenty-first century. On the other hand, being overweight may not be as serious of a risk as being obese. When the definition of overweight was changed from BMI of 27 down to BMI of 25 kg/m^2, the number of people classified as having a health problem dramatically increased. However, it is not clear that those in the range of 25–27 are at greater risk for serious health problems than those who are in the normal weight range. I cannot comment on the esthetic desire to be thin, but for health purposes, being modestly overweight does not appear to be an indication of being "sick."

The Metabolic Syndrome

In addition to long-standing and widely researched diagnoses for diabetes and obesity/overweight, medical and public-health professionals have established a new category of disease called "the metabolic syndrome." This condition is identified by a combination of risk factors, including

- abdominal obesity (defined as excessive fat tissue around the center of the body)
- problematical lipids, characterized by high triglycerides, low HDL cholesterol, and high LDL cholesterol
- modestly elevated blood pressure
- insulin resistance

- high likelihood of blood clotting
- elevation and likelihood of inflammation characterized by c-reactive protein.

People with the metabolic syndrome are at increased risk for heart disease or other diseases associated with the build-up of plaque in the coronary arteries. This syndrome is extremely common. Previously, it was estimated that it affected over 50 million people in the USA. Sometimes, people describe the metabolic syndrome in terms of physical appearance and insulin resistance. People with the syndrome have the appearance of carrying weight in the central parts of their body. This is sometimes described as the "apple" shape (see Fig. 8.9). In addition, the condition is associated with a diabetes-like syndrome of insulin resistance. People with this syndrome are often physically inactive, older, and may have a genetic predisposition. Recently, the definition of the metabolic syndrome changed. The updated criteria for the clinical diagnosis of the metabolic syndrome are summarized in Table 8.2.

Clearly, there is reason to be concerned about the metabolic syndrome. Various studies show that those with the syndrome are at about twice the risk of CVD and at about a five-fold risk of developing diabetes [29]. However, it is less clear that the latest change in the definition of the metabolic syndrome confers additional advantages. Table 8.2 summarized the criteria originally proposed by the World Health Organization in 1998 and the most recent criteria promoted by the American Heart Association and the National Heart, Lung, and Blood Institute. A person can be diagnosed with the

Table 8.2 Definitions for metabolic syndrome according to World Health Organization (1998) and American Heart Association/National Heart Lung, and Blood Institute (2005). The metabolic syndrome requires any three of five clinical abnormalities

Clinical measure	WHO 1998	AHA/NHLBI 2005
Overweight or obese	Waist-to-hip ratio >0.90 for men, >0.85 in women or BMI>30	102 cm (40 inches) in men, 88 cm (35 inches) in women; estimated BMI>25
Elevated triglycerides	>150 mg/dl	150 mg/dl or on drug treatment for elevated triglycerides
Reduced HDL-C	<35 mg/dl in men, <39 mg/dl in women	<40 mg/dl in men, <50 mg/dl in women, or on drug treatment for reduced HDL-C
Elevated blood pressure	>140 mmHg systolic, >90 mmHg diastolic	130 mmHg systolic blood pressure or 85 mmHg diastolic blood pressure or on antihypertensive drug treatment
Elevated fasting glucose	>110 mg/dl	100 mg/dl or on drug treatment for elevated glucose

WHO – World Health Organization
AHA – American Heart Association
NHLBI – National Heart, Lung, and Blood Institute
BMI – Body-Mass Index
HDL-C – High-Density Lipoprotein Cholesterol

metabolic syndrome if he or she has any three of five clinical conditions. Using the recent changes in the definitions, the criteria for being overweight, for HDL-Cholesterol, for high blood pressure, and for high blood sugar have all be relaxed. In addition, the AHA/NHLBI definition substitutes taking mediation for any condition for having clinical evidence of the problem.

Figure 8.10 shows the percentage of the population affected by the metabolic syndrome according to the new criteria. The data are based on analysis of the NHANES [30]. As the figure illustrates, the new definition affects a substantial percentage of the population. By age 50, more than half of the population of the USA has metabolic syndrome and by age 60 more than 60 percent of women have the condition. The scientific statement supporting this new definition did not present any analysis of expected changes in the health outcomes in the population under the new definition. Despite pharmaceutical company-sponsored websites promoting the assessment and the diagnosis of the metabolic syndrome, we have surprisingly little evidence that a diagnosis leads to better patient outcomes.

Not everyone embraces the concept of a metabolic syndrome. Researchers invented the term "metabolic syndrome" to describe the aggregation of cardiovascular risk factors. It was believed that each risk factor was related to insulin resistance. However, the metabolic syndrome was not based on a clear physiological model. Investigators have not been able to show that the individual risk factors, such as high blood pressure, triglycerides, or cholesterol levels, act synergistically. Clinically, each risk factor is treated independently of the others.

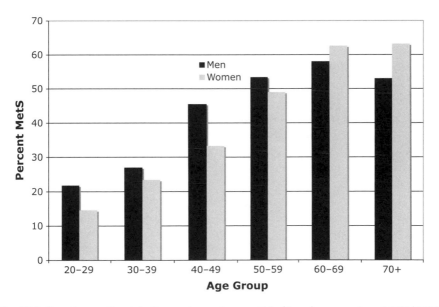

Fig. 8.10 Prevalence of metabolic syndrome in men (*black*) and women (*gray*) NHANES participants. (Adapted from Ford [30].)

Table 8.3 Summary of concerns regarding the metabolic syndrome

1 Criteria are ambiguous or incomplete. Rationale for thresholds are ill defined.
2 Value of including diabetes in the definition is questionable.
3 Insulin resistance as the unifying etiology is uncertain.
4 No clear basis for including/excluding other CVD risk factors.
5 CVD risk value is variable and dependent on the specific risk factors present.
6 The CVD risk associated with the "syndrome" appears to be no greater than the sum of its parts.
7 Treatment of the syndrome is no different than the treatment for each of its components.
8 The medical value of diagnosing the syndrome is unclear.

(From Kahn et al. [31], Table 3.)

Drug treatment for insulin resistance is not available and, with the exception of weight loss, there is not one common treatment. Researchers from the ADA and the European Association for the Study of Diabetes (EASD) have begun to question whether promotion of the concept of a metabolic syndrome has value for patients [31]. A summary of these concerns is listed in Table 8.3. At the end of the day, it is not clear that defining a metabolic syndrome gives us much more information than considering the risk factors independently. Furthermore, we do not know what is gained by the recent modifications in the definition of the metabolic syndrome. More people will get this diagnosis, but will they ultimately be better off because of the new label? At this point, we do not know.

Conclusions

This chapter considered a variety of different topics relevant to the epidemic of obesity in the USA and most western counties. Our waistlines are clearly expanding. As a result, we are becoming increasingly concerned about health problems related to excessive or unnecessary body weight.

Diabetes is clearly the obesity-related health problem that has attracted the most attention, and there is little question that it is a serious health concern. It is a major cause of blindness, kidney failure, heart disease, and amputations. However, in response to concerns about diabetes, a new condition known as "impaired fasting glucose" was created. I could find very little evidence that this newly defined category of illness is positively correlated with the chances of developing diabetes or the complications of diabetes in the future.

The definition "overweight" itself has chanced in recent years. One might say it is now defined as "obesity light." Yet, the older rather than the newer definition of overweight appears more clearly related to poor health outcomes. People included in the new but not the old definition of overweight are no more likely to die prematurely or to have lower quality of life than those in the normal weight category.

Most recently, a new condition known as "the metabolic syndrome" has been defined. Not long after the condition was named, the criteria were broadened to encompass a much larger proportion of the general population. Under the latest definition, most older adults qualify for a diagnosis. As with the other newly defined conditions described in this chapter, there appears to be no clear evidence that the group that qualified only under the newest definition (they would have been excluded under the older definition) are at any greater risk for poor health outcomes. In addition, it remains unclear whether the new definition offers physicians any clear guidance for treatment, beyond what they would know from independently treating the individual risk factors that compose the metabolic syndrome.

In the last three chapters, a common theme has been repeated. New definitions of "disease" have been introduced, and the market for healthcare and expensive interventions has expanded considerably. Yet, we have very little evidence that these definition changes will enhance the health of populations. In the next few chapters, we explore the cost/effectiveness issues relevant to definition changes and consider the requirement that patients become more active in decisions about their own healthcare.

References

1. Association AD. *Diabetes 4-1-1: Facts, Figures, and Statistics at a Glance*. Atlanta: American Diabetes Association; 2006.
2. *Health, United States, 2005*. Atlanta: Centers for Disease Control and Prevention; 2005.
3. Herman WH, Sinnock P, Brenner E, et al. An epidemiologic model for diabetes mellitus: incidence, prevalence, and mortality. *Diabetes Care*. Jul–Aug 1984;7(4):367–371.
4. Knowler WC, Barrett-Connor E, Fowler SE, et al. Reduction in the incidence of type 2 diabetes with lifestyle intervention or metformin. *N Engl J Med*. Feb 7 2002;346(6): 393–403.
5. Harris EL, Wagener DK, Dorman JS, Drash AL. Detection of genetic heterogeneity between families of insulin-dependent diabetes mellitus patients using linkage analysis. *Am J Hum Genet*. Jan 1985;37(1):102–113.
6. Polonsky KS. Dynamics of insulin secretion in obesity and diabetes. *Int J Obes Relat Metab Disord*. Jun 2000;24(Suppl 2):S29–S31.
7. de Luca C, Olefsky JM. Stressed out about obesity and insulin resistance. *Nat Med*. Jan 2006;12(1):41–42; discussion 42.
8. Cavaghan MK, Ehrmann DA, Polonsky KS. Interactions between insulin resistance and insulin secretion in the development of glucose intolerance. *J Clin Invest*. Aug 2000; 106(3):329–333.
9. Report of the Expert Committee on the Diagnosis and Classification of Diabetes Mellitus. *Diabetes Care*. Jul 1997;20(7):1183–1197.
10. Genuth S, Alberti KG, Bennett P, et al. Follow-up report on the diagnosis of diabetes mellitus. *Diabetes Care*. Nov 2003;26(11):3160–3167.
11. Hanefeld M, Temelkova-Kurktschiev T, Schaper F, Henkel E, Siegert G, Koehler C. Impaired fasting glucose is not a risk factor for atherosclerosis. *Diabet Med*. Mar 1999;16(3):212–218.
12. Glucose tolerance and cardiovascular mortality: comparison of fasting and 2-hour diagnostic criteria. *Arch Intern Med*. Feb 12 2001;161(3):397–405.

13. Shaw JE, Zimmet PZ, Hodge AM, et al. Impaired fasting glucose: how low should it go? *Diabetes Care*. Jan 2000;23(1):34–39.
14. Gabir MM, Hanson RL, Dabelea D, et al. The 1997 American Diabetes Association and 1999 World Health Organization criteria for hyperglycemia in the diagnosis and prediction of diabetes. *Diabetes Care*. Aug 2000;23(8):1108–1112.
15. Lorenzo C, Serrano-Rios M, Martinez-Larrad MT, et al. Prevalence of hypertension in Hispanic and non-Hispanic white populations. *Hypertension*. Feb 2002;39(2):203–208.
16. Kaplan RM, Morton D, Wingard DL, Barrett-Connor E. Should the threshold for fasting plasma glucose be reduced: The Rancho Bernardo Study. Unpublished manuscript. 2006.
17. Kanaya AM, Herrington D, Vittinghoff E, et al. Impaired fasting glucose and cardiovascular outcomes in postmenopausal women with coronary artery disease. *Ann Intern Med*. May 17 2005;142(10):813–820.
18. Buchanan TA, Xiang AH, Peters RK, et al. Preservation of pancreatic beta-cell function and prevention of type 2 diabetes by pharmacological treatment of insulin resistance in high-risk hispanic women. *Diabetes*. Sep 2002;51(9):2796–2803.
19. Chiasson JL, Josse RG, Gomis R, Hanefeld M, Karasik A, Laakso M. Acarbose for prevention of type 2 diabetes mellitus: the STOP-NIDDM randomised trial. *Lancet*. Jun 15 2002;359(9323):2072–2077.
20. Pan XR, Li GW, Hu YH, et al. Effects of diet and exercise in preventing NIDDM in people with impaired glucose tolerance. The Da Qing IGT and Diabetes Study. *Diabetes Care*. Apr 1997;20(4):537–544.
21. Tuomilehto J, Lindstrom J, Eriksson JG, et al. Prevention of type 2 diabetes mellitus by changes in lifestyle among subjects with impaired glucose tolerance. *N Engl J Med*. May 3 2001;344(18):1343–1350.
22. Kaplan RM, Ganiats TG, Sieber WJ, Anderson JP. The Quality of Well-Being Scale: critical similarities and differences with SF-36 [see comments]. *Int J Qual Health C*. 1998;10(6):509–520.
23. Kaplan RM, Ganiats TG. Qalys – their ethical implications. *JAMA*. 1990;264(19): 2502–2503.
24. Groessl EJ, Kaplan RM, Barrett-Connor E, Ganiats TG. Body mass index and quality of well-being in a community of older adults. *Am J Prev Med*. Feb 2004;26(2):126–129.
25. Finkelstein EA, Fiebelkorn IC, Wang G. National medical spending attributable to overweight and obesity: how much, and who's paying? *Health Aff (Millwood)*. Jan–Jun 2003;Suppl Web Exclusives:W3-219-226.
26. Finkelstein EA, Ruhm CJ, Kosa KM. Economic causes and consequences of obesity. *Annu Rev Public Health*. 2005;26:239–257.
27. Allison DB, Fontaine KR, Manson JE, Stevens J, VanItallie TB. Annual deaths attributable to obesity in the United States. *JAMA*. Oct 27 1999;282(16):1530–1538.
28. Adams KF, Schatzkin A, Harris TB, et al. Overweight, obesity, and mortality in a large prospective cohort of persons 50 to 71 years old. *N Engl J Med*. Aug 24 2006;355(8): 763–778.
29. Grundy SM, Cleeman JI, Daniels SR, et al. Diagnosis and management of the metabolic syndrome: an American Heart Association/National Heart, Lung, and Blood Institute scientific statement. *Curr Opin Cardiol*. Jan 2006;21(1):1–6.
30. Ford ES. Prevalence of the metabolic syndrome defined by the International Diabetes Federation among adults in the U.S. *Diabetes Care*. Nov 2005;28(11):2745–2749.
31. Kahn R, Buse J, Ferrannini E, Stern M. The metabolic syndrome: time for a critical appraisal: joint statement from the American Diabetes Association and the European Association for the Study of Diabetes. *Diabetes Care*. Sep 2005;28(9):2289–2304.

Chapter 9
Cost-Effectiveness and Opportunity Costs

Are we using our resources wisely in the pursuit of better population health—that is, the general health of our entire population? In order to address this question, we must consider the implications of purchasing healthcare. A good starting point is the comparison of medical decisions and healthcare expenditures in the USA and other countries. While many assume that greater expenditure results in greater health benefit, developed countries that spend considerably less on healthcare in comparison with the USA have about equal health outcomes. Per capita expenditures on healthcare in the UK, for example, are about 40 percent of the per capita expenditures in the USA. As difficult as it may be to believe, life expectancy in the UK is slightly higher than it is in the USA, and infant mortality is slightly lower. Figure 9.1 summarizes life expectancy for men and women in seven countries that participate in the Organization for Economic Development and Cooperation. (OECD is an international organization composed of some 30 mostly developed countries committed to representative democracy and free markets.) Although the USA outspends per capita every one of the six other wealthy countries in the study, both US men and US women have the shortest life expectancies in the group [1].]

It might be argued that spending more on healthcare will result in better-quality healthcare. But even by the roughest measures, this common-sense conclusion does not seem to stand up. Within the USA, there is considerable variability in Medicare spending. For example, data from the Medicare program tell us the per capita expenditure ranges from a low of $2,736 in Oregon to a high of $6,307 in Alaska. State-level data are also available on the average quality of healthcare, typically defined as adherence to defined standards of patient care. For example, it is possible to estimate the extent to which physicians adhere to defined patient guidelines. The association between per capita spending and quality across the USA is shown in Fig. 9.2. As the figure demonstrates, if there is a relationship, it goes in the wrong direction. States that spend more in their Medicare programs appear to do more poorly in indicators of the quality of care they deliver. Adjusting for socioeconomic status does not alter this finding [2].

Many have argued that society has a moral obligation to provide all necessary services for those who are sick and in need of help. Yet, there is no

R.M. Kaplan, *Disease, Diagnoses, and Dollars*, DOI 10.1007/978-0-387-74045-4_9,
© Springer Science+Business Media, LLC 2009

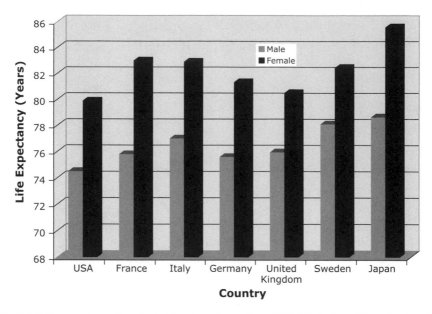

Fig. 9.1 Life expectancy in selected developed courtiers 2005. (Data from Organization for Economic Development and Cooperation.)

assurance that investments in healthcare will improve the general health of the population because many services produce limited benefits. The challenge is in determining how many people are in need of help and whether services will really help them. As discussed in Chapters 5–8, changes in the diagnostic thresholds for diseases have expanded the number of people who are defined as "sick" and therefore considered in need of medical service. This has been accomplished, in part, through screening programs that identify disease in very early phases. At the other extreme, interventions for people who have been neglected and are near death are often both ineffective and expensive. States with very high Medicare costs might be those who fail to attend to poor people until they are near death and then attempt to rescue them with expensive but futile interventions.

Once an individual is identified as "sick," it is incumbent upon the system to treat the problem. We must then ask who gets treatment. Wennberg convincingly demonstrated that individuals with the same conditions receive different services in different geographic areas [3]. To address the inequities and inefficiencies suggested by this finding, evidence-based medicine guidelines, which aim to regularize and standardize diagnosis and treatment procedures, have become a boom industry. And adherence to these guidelines has become the gold standard for quality. For example, in one recent study by McGlynn and colleagues, four nine-member multi-disciplinary panels from different

Relationship Between Quality And Medicare Spending, As Expressed By Overall Quality Ranking, 2000–2001

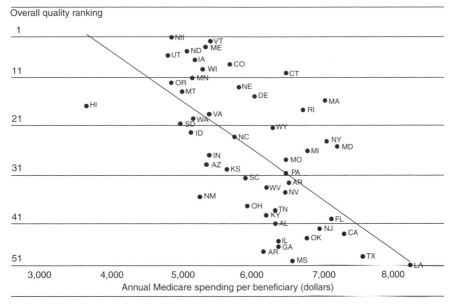

SOURCES: Medicare claims data and S. F. jencks et al., "Change in the Quality of Care Delivered to Medicare Beneficiaries, 1998–1999 to 2000–2001," *Journal of the American Medical Association* 289, no.3 (2003):305–312.
NOTE: For Quality ranking, smaller values equal higher quality.

Fig. 9.2 The relationship between Medicare spending per capita and rank in estimates of quality of care delivered (From Baicker and Chandra [2].)

geographic regions estimated the best approach to the management of a variety of different health conditions. A telephone survey of adults living in 12 metropolitan areas asked about their healthcare experiences and obtained written consent to review their medical records. The investigators evaluated performance on 439 indicators for 30 acute and chronic medical conditions and for preventive care. The study suggested that just more than half the participants received the recommended care for their health conditions. For some conditions, such as alcohol dependence, adherence to recommended care was only about 10 percent. The authors concluded that the health of Americans is compromised because physicians do not adhere to treatment guidelines [4].

As noted in the McGlynn analysis, "poor" quality is defined as failure to do everything identified in the most recent guidelines. However, in many cases, attention to early stages of disease may offer little or no benefit and may even produce harm. Early intervention for prehypertension, IFG, and marginally high levels of LDL cholesterol have now become part of the standard guidelines for care. New proposals that "pay for performance" will financially punish doctors who fail to adhere to these quality standards [5]. Yet, many if not most patients will not benefit from the newly defined approaches to "good" care. Deyo offered examples of adverse "cascade" effects of medical technology. Efforts to screen for or treat mild-spectrum illness often have negative effects and can even cause early death [6], and aggressive approaches to mild-spectrum illness may cause harm by diverting resources away from programs with greater potential benefits for the larger population.

Uninsured Americans: A Result of Too Many Tests?

It is common—and it is human nature—to think of the risks and benefits that medical diagnoses and treatments have at the individual level. But in this book the focus has been on "population health," focusing on the risks and benefits as they apply to large groups of people. In Chapter 5, we considered the benefits of screening for cancer. Most systematic trials show very few benefits for screening women under age 50 for breast cancer. Chapter 6 questioned whether current proposals to create a new disease called prehypertension would actually benefit population health. In Chapter 7, we challenged the belief that most of the population should take statin drugs to reduce their risk for heart disease. In Chapter 8, we considered the benefits of lowering the threshold for the diagnosis of diabetes. Are we, in focusing on the "big picture," going too far? After all, there is very little harm associated with the statin medications. Furthermore, if you or someone in your family had breast cancer would you not want to know? No one is being hurt. Or are they?

There are many arguments in favor of lower disease thresholds and increased screening. One argument is that more people will get treatment early. A second argument is that the risk of new medication seems very small. A third argument is that individuals may have a small chance of benefit, but populations will benefit. Finally, it might be argued that it is not our money anyway. Insurance will pay for the increased costs. So, why should we be concerned?

We do know that increased screening will cause financial problems. Under managed care, it is difficult to deny a service for a "peer-defined diagnosis," meaning a diagnosis officially defined by a reputable board of medical experts. For example, consider the recommendations of the American Cancer Society, the hypertension standard contained in JNC-7, ATP III's recommendations on cholesterol screening, and the disease definitions put forth by the Committee on Diagnosis and Classification of Diabetes. Official pronouncements like these have all suggested more aggressive approaches to treatment, and once these standards have been made public, managed-care institutions are very unlikely to deny the recommended treatments or other procedures. The economic forces at work are not all that hard to understand. Managed-care groups are likely to be sued if someone dies or develops a serious disability from a condition for which screening was recommended but not performed. It is certain, for example, people will continue to have strokes, heart attacks, and breast cancer. If a patient is denied screening for these problems and eventually develops the illness, a lawsuit is highly probable. And the suit is likely to be successful, even though the evidence suggests that the patient would not have been better off had they been screened. Managed care, in effect, is going to be responsible for covering "pseudodisease."

In analyzing a particular program of spending or investment, economists often talk of the "opportunity cost." Roughly speaking, this is the cost of other opportunities foregone whenever you make a particular economic choice to spend or invest. For example, if a town chooses to build a playground on a piece of its land instead of selling the land or leasing it, the money not earned from the sale or lease is an opportunity cost.

The opportunity-cost problems that arise in major population health decisions suggest that large numbers of people will be harmed by the additional expenses incurred by downwardly revised diagnostic thresholds or broader disease definitions. These changes in definitions and thresholds often drive investment and expenditure into previously untreated segments of the population, and when that happens, some other previously funded segment is likely to see its level of expenditure or investment decrease. Put more bluntly, if the pool of diseased individuals is enlarged, so will the expense, and that means something is got to give is best illustrated in an analysis recently reported by Gilmer and Kronick, summarized in Fig. 9.3. The graph traces the relationship between per capita health expenditure and the percentage of workers who are uninsured. Between 1979 and 2002, these two variables track almost perfectly. To adjust for inflation, per capita healthcare expenditure is divided by median income. As the figure suggests, these increases in the cost of health insurance are very highly associated with the percentage of the workforce that is uninsured. Changes in disease thresholds and increases in screening make healthcare costs go up. Increased healthcare costs are passed on to employers as higher insurance premiums. Each time the premiums go up, more employers decide not to insure their workers. As a result, the percentage of uninsured systematically increases.

Changes in disease thresholds may have relatively little effect on population health for insured patients. On the other hand, threshold changes may negatively affect many other people. More services for well-insured people may lead to higher healthcare costs, which in turn may lead to increases in the number of people who have no health insurance at all (either because they cannot afford it or because it is not offered to them). Uninsured and underinsured people are the most likely to suffer from such broad reductions in services. In other words, promoting the use of ineffective health services for the well-insured fortunate might have the unintended consequence of lowering general population health, with most of the burden borne by those least able to afford it.

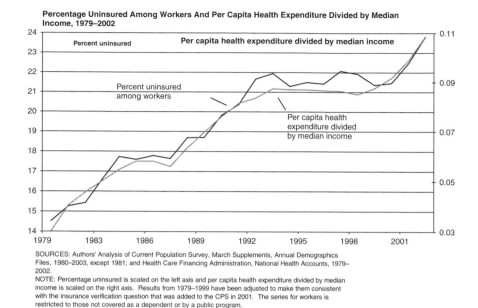

Fig. 9.3 Percentage of uninsured workers and per capita healthcare expenditures divided by the median income: 1979–2002. (From Gilmer and Kronick, 2005. [7])

The Costs of Care

The treatment of the newly defined illness has become expensive. Pharmaceutical costs are now one of the strongest drivers of increases in healthcare costs. Pharmaceutical costs rose twice as fast as other components of healthcare expenditures during the 1990 s. In the first few years of the twenty-first century, the costs of prescription medications for Medicare patients were rising about 20 percent each year. For most chronic conditions, an expensive pharmaceutical product is available with treatment costs approaching $3 per day. For older adults with multiple diagnoses, the costs of medications often exceed the cost of food [8].

In order to attack problems in the allocation of health resources, we need models that will help us think through the alternatives. The remainder of this chapter offers a model to guide public policy decisions.

Outcomes in Chronic Illness

One of the most important things a healthcare model does is to define a unit of benefit. The traditional healthcare model usually links a benefit to a particular diagnosis. For example, an outcome might be assessed by changes in blood pressure, to tumor size, or to death from a heart attack. To take just one instance of diagnosis-linked benefit measurement, contemporary preventive cardiology care is based on observations from the coronary primary prevention trial (CPPT) [9, 10]. In this experimental trial, men were randomly assigned to take either a placebo or use a drug known as cholestyrmanine. Cholestyrmanine can significantly lower serum cholesterol and, in this particular trial, produced an average total cholesterol reduction of 8.5 percent. In comparison to men using a placebo, men in the treatment group experienced 24 percent fewer heart-attack deaths and 19 percent fewer non-fatal heart attacks. So, the benefit of taking the medication was linked to a particular diagnosis, namely heart attack.

The CPPT was reviewed in Chapter 7, where it was noted that there was a 24-percent reduction in cardiovascular mortality in the treated group in comparison with those who took a placebo. The absolute proportion of patients who died of CVD was similar in the two groups. In the placebo group, there were 38 deaths among 1,900 participants (2 percent). In the cholestyrmanine group there were 30 deaths among 1,906 participants (1.6 percent). In other words, taking medication for 6 years reduced the chances of dying from CVD from 2 percent to 1.6 percent. However, the diagnosis-specific medical model focuses on cardiovascular deaths because the medicine was designed to reduce deaths from heart disease. Considering all causes of death, there was essentially no benefit of treatment. At the end of the study, 3.7 percent of those in the placebo group had died and 3.6 percent of those in the cholestyrmanine group had died. Since the publication of the CPPT, several other studies have obtained similar results. Cholesterol- lowering may reduce the chances of dying of heart disease, but it does not always reduce the chances of dying prematurely.

An alternative way of looking at the same data, using an outcomes model, does not take cause of death into consideration. From the outcomes perspective, the focus is on whether the patient is alive [11]. In Chapter 5, a similar analysis applied to cancer screening. Although cancer-screening tests may reduce the chances that people die from breast or colon cancer, randomized trials typically fail to show that screening extends life expectancy. If a medication or a test reduces the chances of dying from one disease while increasing the chances of dying from another, it is most likely not meeting the original objectives of the patient [12]. Since, virtually all treatments have the potential to produce harm as well as benefit, the outcomes model may be the most appropriate to evaluate benefits of treatment.

Mortality

Public-health statistics concentrate on death rates. One major indicator is life expectancy, defined as the median number of years of life expected for each birth cohort. The second major indicator is infant mortality, which is defined as the number of babies born alive that die within 1 year. Infant mortality is usually expressed per 100,000 live births. Mortality remains the major outcome measure in most epidemiological studies and clinical trials.

Obviously, any model of health outcome that excluded mortality would be incomplete. Indeed, many public-health statistics focus exclusively on mortality through estimates of crude mortality rates, age-adjusted mortality rates, and infant mortality rates. However, many significant health conditions are not well reflected by mortality information. For example, osteoarthritis, cataract disease, and minor depression may all cause poor health without affecting life expectancy or infant mortality statistics.

Health-Related Quality of Life

How to conceptualize and measure health status on a large scale—that is, as population health—has been a concern of scholars for many decades. In his influential 1958 book "The Affluent Society," John Kenneth Galbraith described the need to measure the effect of the healthcare system on "quality of life" [13]. At the end of the Eisenhower administration, a President's Commission on National Goals identified health status measurement as an important objective. Within a few years, Galbraith's idea and the impetus provided by the presidential commission prompted the first formal and quantifiable measures of quality of life as an indicator of health status.

Sullivan (1966) argued that behavioral indicators such as absenteeism, bed-disability days, and institutional confinement were the most important consequences of disease and disability. Ability to perform activities (such as walking unassisted, climbing stairs, writing, dialing a telephone number, doing basic arithmetic) at different ages could be compared to societal standards for these behaviors, so that standards could be age-adjusted. Restrictions in usual activity were seen as prima facie evidence of deviation from well-being. Health conditions affect behavior and, in this chapter, health outcomes are conceptualized as observable behavioral consequences of a health state [14]. Arthritis, for example, may be associated with difficulty in walking, observable limping, or problems in using the hands. Even a minor illness, such as the common cold, might result in disruptions in daily activities, alterations in activity patterns, and decreased work capacity. Think back to your most recent illness. Arthritis may have limited your ability to climb stairs or to play tennis. Your common cold, although brief, may have disrupted your work or your social life. These disruptions in life activities caused by illness represent losses in health-related quality of life.

Although they are obviously important as health indicators, life expectancy and infant mortality ignore the morbidity or dysfunction people may suffer while they are still alive. The National Center for Health Statistics, part of the Centers for Disease Control and Prevention, addressed this shortcoming by providing information and standard definitions for a variety of states of morbidity. For example, it defined "disability" as a temporary or long-term reduction in a person's activity. Over the last 30 years, medical- and health-service researchers have refined and elaborated the definitions and standards so that health-status assessments can be stated quantitatively. These standards are often called "quality of life" measures, but because they are used exclusively to evaluate health status, we prefer the more descriptive phrase "health-related quality of life" [15]. Some approaches to the measurement of health-related quality of life combine measures of morbidity and mortality to express health outcomes in units analogous to years of life. The years of life figure, however, is adjusted for diminished quality of life associated with diseases or disabilities [16].

Modern measures of health outcome consider future as well as current health status. Cancer, for example, may have very little impact on current functioning but may have a substantial impact on behavioral outcomes in the future. Today, a person with a malignant tumor in a leg may be functioning very much like a person with a leg muscle injury. However, the cancer patient is more likely to remain dysfunctional in the future. Comprehensive expressions of health status need to incorporate estimates of future behavioral dysfunction as well as to measure current status [17].

The spectrum of medical care ranges from public health, preventive medicine, and environmental control through diagnosis to therapeutic intervention, convalescence, and rehabilitation. Many programs affect the probability of occurrence of future dysfunction, rather than altering present functional status. In many aspects of preventive care, for example, the benefit of the treatment cannot be seen until many years after the intervention. A supportive family that instills proper health habits in its children, for example, may also promote better health in the future, even though the benefit may not be realized for years. As mentioned above, the concept of health must consider not only a person's current ability to function but also the probability of future changes in function or probabilities of death. A person who is very functional and asymptomatic today may harbor a disease with a poor prognosis. For example, many individuals are at high risk of dying from heart disease even though they are perfectly functional today. Should we call them "healthy?" The term "severity of illness" should take into consideration both dysfunction and prognosis. Comprehensive models that combine morbidity, mortality, and prognosis have been described in the literature [17]. A behavioral conceptualization of health status can represent this prognosis by modeling disruptions in behavior that might occur in the future [12].

Opportunity Costs

So far we have concentrated on controversies about the effects of screening on health outcomes. Although some are skeptical about the benefits of testing, others have argued that the tests rarely harm patients. The PSA is a simple blood draw and, although unpleasant, sigmoidoscopy and colonoscopy rarely result in perforated colons. Why not continue to test everyone? Perhaps the most important reason is that screening adds significant cost to healthcare. There are subtle differences between how economists use the word "cost" and how it is used more generally. Most people think of cost in terms of dollars. However, economists try not to place value judgments on decisions. Instead, they attempt to identify the alternatives and to spell out the consequences of various choices. Opportunity costs, as briefly described above, are opportunities forgone when resources are used to support a particular decision. To consider an example of an opportunity cost that arises when we make health-care decisions, think of what happens when we as a society spend a lot of money on screening. Simply put, what happens is there will be less money to spend on other healthcare programs.

A wide variety of analyses have evaluated cancer-screening tests using a metric of cost per QALY produced. Some programs, such as pap smears for older low-income women, save both money and lives [18]. On the other hand, screening for prostate cancer with either digital rectal exams or PSA both drain resources and could cause harm [19]. The harm occurs when someone with only a small potential to gain health from treatment is exposed to the risks of treatment and further testing. For example, treatment of prostate cancer in older men may have little potential to extend life or improve life quality. However, the treatment might cause reduced quality of life because it results in incontinence, impotence, or impaired bowel function. In many cases, cancer screening does produce some benefit. However, it is a very expensive use of resources in relation to many other alternatives. For example, lifelong screening with chest X-ray for skin thickness and local cutaneous melanoma may produce a benefit, but at a cost of $250,000 per QALY [20]. Programs such as smoking prevention produce a QALY for less that $1,000. In other words, 250 smoking prevention programs might be funded for the cost of one chest X-ray-screening program. Put another way, the population health benefit of funding smoking prevention may be 250 times greater.

Comparing programs for a given population with a given medical condition, cost-effectiveness is measured as the change in costs of care for the program compared with the existing therapy or program, relative to the change in health measured in a standardized unit such as the QALY. The difference in costs over the difference in effectiveness is the incremental cost-effectiveness and is usually expressed as the cost/QALY. Since the objective of all programs is to produce QALYs, the cost/QALY ratio can be used to show the relative efficiency of different programs [21].

There have been several cost/utility analyses of cholesterol screening and treatment. Goldman and colleagues [22] modeled the value of screening for high cholesterol and treatment with the latest statins or HMG CoA reductase inhibitor (in this case lovastatin). Their model considered recurrent heart attack rates using data from the Framingham Heart Study. One simulation considered men with total cholesterol values in excess of 300 mg/dl but no other risk factors for heart disease. For these men, the cost to produce a year of life was estimated to be between $71,000 and $135,000. For women, estimates ranged from $84,000 to $390,000 per life year. If the threshold for initiating treatment is lowered to 250 mg/dl, the cost to produce a year of life

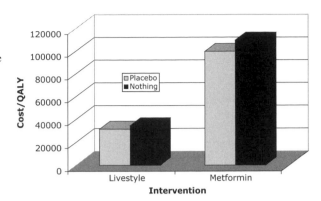

Fig. 9.4 Cost/QALY of lifestyle and metformin in the Diabetes Prevention Program estimated using the health system perspective

increases to between $105,000 and $270,000 for men. Recent campaigns have attempted to increase the number of adults on treatment. Until recently, the threshold for a diagnosis of hypercholesterolemia was 240 mg/dl. Under that definition, about 1 in 5 adults qualified. With the more recent push toward defining high cholesterol as greater than 200 mg/dl, about half of all adults will be deemed abnormal [23]. However, the lower the diagnostic threshold, the less the cost-effectiveness of screening and treatment will be.

Simulations of the cost-effectiveness of heart-disease prevention have been reported by Prosser and colleagues. These investigators used the Harvard Policy Model to estimate the cost-effectiveness of cholesterol-lowering therapies for adults with different risk factors. Using an established model, they simulated benefits of treatments for men and women aged 35–84. The simulation included LDL cholesterol levels greater than 160 mg/dl. Overall, the model considered 240 risk subgroups stratified by age, sex, and presence of risk factors. The risk factors included in the model were smoking status, blood pressure, LDL cholesterol, and HDL cholesterol. Taking a societal perspective and using a 30-year time horizon, the analysis demonstrated that the cost-effectiveness of primary prevention for low-risk adults using diet therapy was less than $100,000/QALY. However, the cost-effectiveness for secondary prevention using a statin medication was as high as $420,000/QALY for men and $1,400,000/QALY for women.

Primary-Prevention Approaches

Healthcare professionals make a distinction between primary and secondary prevention measures. Primary prevention requires action before disease has reached the accepted diagnostic or clinical threshold. Typically, primary prevention involves lifestyle and behavioral changes (including diet and exercise) rather than explicitly medical (pharmaceutical or surgical or procedural) interventions. Secondary prevention involves intervention once the disease process begins. For example, treating high cholesterol with a statin drug or managing high blood pressure with medication are examples of secondary prevention. The treatments are used to prevent the established disease from resulting in a bad outcome like a heart attack or a stroke.

When planning population-health strategies, both primary and secondary prevention strategies should be considered. Health care officials are typically enthusiastic about supporting secondary prevention in the form of screening programs and treatments for high cholesterol or high blood pressure. Primary prevention programs usually get less consideration. Three of the most successful primary prevention programs are smoking cessation, injury control, and increased physical activity. For the balance of this chapter we will discuss just one program—physical activity.

Physical Activity

Research shows that people who are physically active live significantly longer than those who are sedentary [24]. These studies have documented a relationship between physical activity and all-causes mortality, CHD mortality, mortality from diabetes mellitus, and mortality associated with cystic fibrosis and other diseases. In addition to living longer, those who engage in regular physical activity may be better able to perform the normal activities of daily living and enjoy many aspects of life not available to the inactive adult. Furthermore, those who exercise regularly have better insulin sensitivity and less abdominal obesity [25]. Regular exercise has been shown to improve psychological well-being for those with mood disorders [26]. Some evidence has even suggested that the costs of poor health outcomes associated with physical inactivity exceed those attributable to obesity, hypertension, and smoking [27]. The Centers for Disease Control estimate that physical inactivity is the most common among risk factors for heart disease and carries a greater population-attributable risk than high cholesterol or hypertension. Successful programs have been developed to promote exercise for the general population [28]. Furthermore, specific interventions have been developed for those diagnosed with particular diseases [29].

Despite the benefits of exercise, few people will start an exercise program, and many of those who start do not continue to exercise [30]. Some predictors of failure to exercise regularly include being overweight, low socio-economic status, female gender, television watching and smoking [31]. However, the most commonly reported barriers to exercise are lack of time and inaccessibility of facilities. Studies show that exercise patterns change as people age. Physical activity begins to decline by late childhood and the downward trend accelerates in the late teens and early twenties [32]. It appears that Americans are shifting toward less vigorous activity patterns, with walking becoming the most common form of exercise. Physical inactivity is increasing as Americans spend more time watching television or working with computers [33].

In order to estimate the cost/utility of exercise programs, Hatziandreu et al. [34] developed a simulation model. This computer model created two hypothetical cohorts of 35-year-old men and followed them for 30 years. The model was calculated for 1,000 men assumed to jog regularly and another 1,000 men assumed to be inactive. In addition to the health benefits of exercise, negative effects were subtracted from the benefits. These include injuries and low adherence. Costs included running equipment, treating injuries, and the value of the time spent exercising. The costs of treating heart disease for those estimated to be affected were also included. The analysis showed that jogging reduces heart disease, so money is saved for those who exercise regularly. The analysis suggested that regular exercise produces a QALY for about $11,313. In other words, the cost to produce a year of life is quite low relative to most medical and secondary prevention efforts.

Another example of the benefits of lifestyle interventions comes from a study of the prevention of type 2 diabetes. Type 2 diabetes is the most common form of the condition. It typically starts after age 40, and it is highly associated with being obese or overweight. Perhaps attributable to the increasing rate of overweight in youth, type 2 is starting to emerge as a common health problem in younger people. The goal of the diabetes prevention program [35] was to prevent transition to type 2 diabetes in patients who were identified as at risk. These at-risk volunteers were randomly assigned to one of three conditions: intensive lifestyle modification, metformin (an oral drug that lowers blood sugar), or placebo. The DPP included 3,234 adults with impaired glucose tolerance. The intensive lifestyle intervention was designed to reduce the initial body weight by 7 percent through regular physical activity and diet. The metformin group took one 850-mg tablet each day. The placebo group also took one tablet per day. The patients were evaluated before randomization and at yearly intervals over the course of 3 years.

Quality of life was measured using the Quality of Well-being Scale (QWB). The measure was chosen because it can be used to estimate QALYs. Over the course of 3 years, those randomly assigned to the lifestyle intervention accrued 0.050 more QALYs than those assigned a regular dose of metformin. Among the three interventions, the lifestyle approach was the most expensive (total cost US $27,065 in 2,000). Metformin was less expensive ($25,937), while the placebo was the least expensive option ($23,525). Figure 9.5 summarizes the cost/QALY for the lifestyle and the metformin conditions from a healthcare system perspective. The figure shows the cost/QALY attributable to the interventions in comparison to placebo and in comparison to doing nothing. Although both interventions offer significant benefits over placebo or doing nothing, the cost/QALY for the lifestyle invention was significantly lower than that for metformin. In other words, even though the lifestyle intervention was more expensive, it offers significantly better value for money.

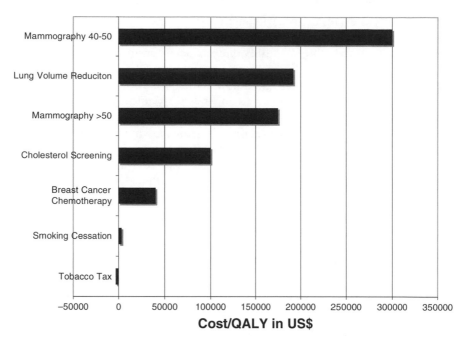

Fig. 9.5 Graphic League Table analysis of Cost/QALY for several programs. The tobacco tax actually saves money. A support program to assist with weight loss produces a QALY at a low cost, while lung volume reduction surgery for emphysema produces QALYs, but at a very high cost.

Leagu Table

Policies advocating changes in diagnostic thresholds will almost certainly add to healthcare costs. In order to evaluate whether these decisions are wise uses of resources, analysts have used "league tables" that compare the cost utility of these decisions versus alternative uses of the scarce healthcare resources these decisions consume. Using the available literature on the cost/QALY for various medical and public-health interventions, we need to estimate the policy consequences of treating patients who have mild-spectrum problems. For example, the cost/QALY for treating some mild-spectrum condition might be $800,000/QALY. Using resources to screen and treat this hypothetical condition might reduce the opportunity to support a program that produces a QALY for $50,000. In other words, each QALY gained by pursuing mild-spectrum conditions might take resources away from a program that could produce 16 QALYs at the same cost.

Figure 9.5 summarizes the cost/QALY for several programs. The figure is a graphic representation of a league table. Some approaches to enhancing public health, such as tobacco taxes, actually raise money while offering population health benefits. Other approaches, such as chemotherapy for breast cancer, are intermediate in the cost/QALY, while surgical interventions for advanced emphysema (estimated from the National Emphysema Treatment Trial-NETT) also produce QALYs at a very high cost. If our goal is to make the population healthy, we might want to use cost/QALY as a guide to resource allocation.

Summary

Healthcare interventions have costs, risks, and benefits. Lowering the diagnostic thresholds for common heart-disease risk factors is likely to benefit the population. However, not all people will benefit equally. People at the highest risk levels will benefit most, and those lower on the risk spectrum will gain much less benefit. Costs, on the other hand, will accrue to people at all levels of the disease spectrum. Although costs are expected to be higher for those most at risk, those with only mild risk will also face significant and recurring expenses.

The costs of changing disease thresholds may have more general consequences—not limited to heart disease, and affecting not just an individual's health and healthcare expense. New definitions of disease will be associated with higher average healthcare costs across large populations. Evidence suggests that employers, when confronted with higher costs, are more likely to stop providing healthcare for their workforce. Between 1979 and 2002, the number of uninsured almost perfectly tracked the costs of providing healthcare to employees. High healthcare costs mean that more people will face the consequences of having no reliable and affordable source of healthcare. Among the uninsured, many serious and treatable illnesses may be overlooked. In other words, the luxury of treating mild-spectrum illness may have only marginal benefits for those fortunate enough to be covered. But the consequence may be higher healthcare costs, and ultimately an increased chance of harm to those left uninsured or underinsured because their employers refused to keep up with the escalating costs.

There are other options. Lifestyle interventions are recommended in most guidelines. Studies suggested that lifestyle programs are a better use of resources than wide-scale use of medicines. A prudent diet and regular exercise program may help prevent heart disease. In addition, these same lifestyle changes may contribute to a reduction in the risks of cancer, diabetes, and several other chronic conditions. Furthermore, they may contribute to a better appearance and a greater level of energy. High priced pharmaceutical products should be considered as an options when lifestyle fails, not as a first line of defense.

This chapter has considered some policy options for controlling costs and achieving better health outcomes. In Chapter 10, we will explore in greater detail options for individual patients.

References

1. Starfield B. Is US health really the best in the world? *JAMA*. 2000;284(4):483–485.
2. Baicker K, Chandra A. Medicare spending, the physician workforce, and beneficiaries' quality of care. *Health Aff (Millwood)*. 2004;Suppl Web Exclusive:W184–W197.
3. Wennberg JE, Fisher ES, Skinner JS. Geography and the debate over Medicare reform. *Health Aff (Millwood)*. 2002;Suppl Web Exclusives:W96–W114.
4. McGlynn EA, Asch SM, Adams J, et al. The quality of health care delivered to adults in the United States. *N Engl J Med*. Jun 26 2003;348(26):2635–2645.
5. Dolinar RO, Leininger SL. Pay for performance means compliance-based care. *J Am Med Dir Assoc*. Jun 2006;7(5):328–333.
6. Deyo RA. Cascade effects of medical technology. *Annu Rev Public Health*. 2002;23:23–44.
7. Gilmer T, Kronick R. It's the premiums, stupid: projections of the uninsured through 2013. *Health Aff (Millwood)* 2005.
8. Liberman A, Rubinstein J. Health care reform and the pharmaceutical industry: crucial decisions are expected. *Health Care Manag (Frederick)*. Mar 2002;20(3):22–32.
9. The Lipid Research Clinics Coronary Primary Prevention Trial results. I. Reduction in incidence of coronary heart disease. *JAMA*. 1984;251(3):351–364.
10. The Lipid Research Clinics Coronary Primary Prevention Trial results. II. The relationship of reduction in incidence of coronary heart disease to cholesterol lowering. *JAMA*. 1984;251(3):365–374.
11. Golomb BA. Cholesterol and violence: is there a connection? [see comments]. *Ann Intern Med*. 1998;128(6):478–487.
12. Kaplan RM. Behavior as the central outcome in health care. *Am Psychol*. 1990;45(11): 1211–1220.
13. Galbraith JK. *The Affluent Society*. Boston: Houghton Mifflin; 1958.
14. Sullivan DF. Conceptual problems in developing an index of health. Washington: US Dept. of Health Education and Welfare Public Health Service; 1966.
15. Kaplan RM, Bush JW. Health-related quality of life measurement for evaluation research and policy analysis. *Health Psychol*. 1982;1(1):1–20.
16. Kaplan RM, Alcaraz JE, Anderson JP, Weisman M. Quality-adjusted life years lost to arthritis: effects of gender, race, and social class. *Arthrit Care Res*. 1996;9(6):473–482.
17. Kaplan RM. The Ziggy theorem: toward an outcomes-focused health psychology. *Health Psychol*. 1994;13(6):451–460.
18. Fahs M, Mandelblatt J. Cost-effectiveness of cervical cancer screening among elderly low-income women. In: Goldbloom R, Lawrence R, eds. *Preventing Disease: Beyond the Rhetoric*. New York: Springer-Verlag; 1990:441–446.
19. Krahn MD, Mahoney JE, Eckman MH, Trachtenberg J, Pauker SG, Detsky AS. Screening for prostate cancer: a decision analytic view. *JAMA*. Sep 14 1994;272(10):773–780.
20. Mooney MM, Mettlin C, Michalek AM, Petrelli NJ, Kraybill WG. Life-long screening of patients with intermediate-thickness cutaneous melanoma for asymptomatic pulmonary recurrences: a cost-effectiveness analysis. *Cancer*. Sep 15 1997;80(6):1052–1064.
21. Kaplan R, Anderson J. The general health policy model: an integrated approach. In: Spilker B, ed. *Quality of Life and Pharmacoeconomics in Clinical Trials*. New York: Raven; 1996:309–322.
22. Goldman L, Weinstein MC, Goldman PA, Williams LW. Cost-effectiveness of HMG-CoA reductase inhibition for primary and secondary prevention of coronary heart disease. *JAMA*. Mar 6 1991;265(9):1145–1151.
23. Fisher ES, Welch HG. Avoiding the unintended consequences of growth in medical care: how might more be worse? *JAMA* 1999;281:446-453.
24. Warburton DE, Nicol CW, Bredin SS. Health benefits of physical activity: the evidence. *CMAJ*. Mar 14 2006;174(6):801–809.

25. Misra A, Alappan NK, Vikram NK, et al. Effect of supervised progressive resistance-exercise training protocol on insulin sensitivity, glycemia, lipids, and body composition in Asian Indians with type 2 diabetes. *Diabetes Care* 2008;31:1282–1287.
26. Netz Y, Zach S, Taffe JR, Guthrie J, Dennerstein L. Habitual physical activity is a meaningful predictor of well-being in mid-life women: a longitudinal analysis. *Climacteric* 2008;11:337–344.
27. Oldridge NB. Economic burden of physical inactivity: healthcare costs associated with cardiovascular disease. *Eur J Cardiovasc Prev Rehabil* 2008;15:130–139.
28. Muller-Riemenschneider F, Reinhold T, Nocon M, Willich SN. Long-term effectiveness of interventions promoting physical activity: A systematic review. *Prev Med* 2008.
29. McAndrew LM, Musumeci-Szabo TJ, Mora PA, et al. Using the common sense model to design interventions for the prevention and management of chronic illness threats: from description to process. *Br J Health Psychol* 2008;13:195–204.
30. Dishman RK, Saunders RP, Motl RW, Dowda M, Pate RR. Self-efficacy moderates the relation between declines in physical activity and perceived social support in high school girls. *J Pediatr Psychol* 2008.
31. Boutelle KN, Jeffery RW, French SA. Predictors of vigorous exercise adoption and maintenance over four years in a community sample. *Int J Behav Nutr Phys Act* 2004;1:13.
32. Troiano RP, Berrigan D, Dodd KW, Masse LC, Tilert T, McDowell M. Physical activity in the United States measured by accelerometer. *Med Sci Sports Exerc* 2008;40:181–188.
33. Singh GK, Kogan MD, Siahpush M, van Dyck PC. Independent and joint effects of socioeconomic, behavioral, and neighborhood characteristics on physical inactivity and activity levels among US children and adolescents. *J Community Health* 2008;33:206–216.
34. Hatziandreu EI, Koplan JP, Weinstein MC, Caspersen CJ, Warner KE. A cost-effectiveness analysis of exercise as a health promotion activity. *Am J Public Health* 1988;78:1417–1421.
35. Within-trial cost-effectiveness of lifestyle intervention or metformin for the primary prevention of type 2 diabetes. *Diabetes Care*. Sep 2003;26(9):2518–2523.

Chapter 10
Shared Medical Decision-Making

I have heard two different complaints from members of my family about the discussions they have had with their doctors. During her advanced years, my mother often complained that her doctor never asked about her preferences for alternative treatments. "Too busy," she noted. The doctor would report, "We are going to put you on a new medicine." Who did he mean by "we"? At the other extreme, my brother noted that his doctor once explained that there were many different approaches for his problem and threw up his hands because he did not know which one was best. My brother asked, "Which one would you use on yourself?"—and they went with that alternative. Neither of these stories is likely to inspire much faith or confidence in how the medical decision-making process works. In both cases, which I believe are not atypical, the patient's preferences were not appropriately assessed.

The Institute of Medicine of the National Academies of Science has issued a series of reports on quality in medicine. Two components of high-quality medicine, according to the report, are that decisions are based on the best research evidence, and that decisions are patient-centered. Chapters 5–8 of this book questioned the evidence base for recent changes in treatment guidelines and disease definitions, and hinted at the idea that many treatments are oversold to patients. In this chapter, we examine this idea of overselling more closely, and question the extent to which modern medicine is patient-centered and offers approaches for patients to become more involved in their own medical decisions.

Uncertainty in Medicine

Throughout the history of medicine, patients have depended on the advice of their doctors, and today most people still believe that "the doctor knows best" [1]. However, over the last few years, newer approaches to medical decision-making have developed. One of the most important movements is called shared decision-making, which involves a two-way exchange between patients and physicians. It is an appropriate decision-making model because there is so

R.M. Kaplan, *Disease, Diagnoses, and Dollars*, DOI 10.1007/978-0-387-74045-4_10,   149
© Springer Science+Business Media, LLC 2009

much uncertainty about many medical choices. An absolutely clear course of action is not known for most medical problems. Treatment alternatives have risks and benefits. In order to approach these uncertainties, we must learn something about patients' tolerance for risk or their willingness to cope with some of the undesirable consequences of treatment. Shared decision-making requires involvement of both the physician and the patient. In some cases, others might be involved, including family members [2].

Shared Decision-Making

Chapters 5–8 argued that decisions about screening for cancer and heart-disease risk factors are very difficult. A test may be accurate in detecting a condition for which there is no effective therapy. Unless the disease can be successfully treated, early detection, compliance with medication programs, and other medical interventions make little difference. Even for tests that lead to effective treatments, undesirable side effects must also be taken into consideration. Russell, in her controversial book "*Educated Guesses*," [3] argued that the use of screening tests is based on informed guesses about the likelihood of benefit. After reviewing a series of tests, she concluded that educated guesses support current policy to screen for high cholesterol and prostate cancer. However, there is equally good evidence supporting educated guesses that these same tests should *not* be used. We have relatively little evidence that new guidelines defining lower diagnostic thresholds for blood pressure, cholesterol, or blood sugar will benefit most patients. To date, few trials have evaluated treatments in patients with mild-spectrum illness. Nevertheless, we are willing to label patients who elect not to use these tests as "noncompliant."

In order to address the issue of how to make decisions in a world of ambiguous or incomplete evaluations, we need greater disclosure of the uncertainties surrounding the use of some tests. When the evidence is uncertain, the uncertainty should be shared with the patients, and patients should be involved in the decision process. The traditional biomedical model continues to emphasize the find-it-fix-it approach. It fails to recognize that detection of disease sometimes leads to little or no patient benefit. Chapter 5 described the 1997 National Cancer Institute (NCI) review of screening mammography for women between the ages of 40 and 49. The NCI thought the panel would support recommendations to screen 40-year-olds. However, after carefully considering the evidence, the panel voted 10 to 2 to be more cautious. Their report stated:

The data currently available did not warrant a universal recommendation for mammography for all women in their forties. Each woman should decide for herself whether to undergo mammography .... given both the importance and complexity of the issues involved in assessing the evidence, a woman should have access to the best possible relevant information regarding both benefits and risks, presented in an understandable and useable form. [NIH consensus statement, 1997].

The suggestion that patients should be involved in the decision process was regarded as shocking by the media, and the members of the review group were accused of committing fraud despite the fact that their recommendation was consistent with virtually every other scientific review of the evidence [4]. One nightly news program began their telecast with an apology to American women for the panel's report [5]. Two weeks later, Senator Kaye Bailey Hutchison (R-Texas) introduced a resolution in the Senate declaring that the panel's conclusion was based on factual errors and that women in their forties should be screened for breast cancer using mammography. The Senate approved the resolution by a vote of 98-0 [6].

Perhaps most disturbing is the reaction to what the report actually said. The committee concluded that women should have access to the best possible information about the risks and benefits of screening and they should make their own decisions. These decisions are not inconsequential. For example, evidence suggests that women between the ages of 40 and 50 who begin getting regular mammograms have essentially no greater likelihood of avoiding death from breast cancer than women who do not get screened regularly (see Chapter 5). However, about one-third of these women will have a false-positive test that requires additional evaluation [7]. Among women who do not have breast cancer, an estimated 18.6 percent will undergo biopsy after ten mammograms and about 6 percent of those who have regular clinical breast exams, but do not have cancer, will get painful and invasive biopsies [8]. A German analysis by Porzsolt and colleagues found that death resulting from breast cancer could be prevented in 6 of 1,000 women who get regular mammography and 5 of 1,000 women who do not get mammography [9]. The traditional biomedical model argues that women should be advised to get mammograms, and that those who fail to do so should get assistance for their non-compliance. In the past, the risks and benefits were rarely discussed. A growing movement suggests all information should be disclosed and that the decision about screening should be shared between the provider and the patient.

There are many other examples of the need for shared medical decision-making. For example, in 1916, obstetricians suggested that women who had given birth by cesarean section should have this surgical procedure repeated for each later birth. This policy dominated obstetrics for the next 70 years. However, in 1984, the American College of Obstetrics and Gynecology encouraged women to have a trial of labor before a cesarean section if they had a low transverse uterine scar. A systematic review of 292 articles by a consensus group suggested that neither alternative is clearly advantageous. Women who have a trial of labor may be at increased risk for uterine rupture, although the probability of this event is quite low (0.24 percent). Elective repeat cesarean section may be associated with greater risks of infection and bleeding. Infant outcomes appear equivalent with either method of delivery except for those few infants with APGAR scores less than 7. After reviewing literature, Roberts and colleagues argued that the choice between these alternatives should be made by the informed woman, not her doctor [10]. The role of the doctor is to help the woman make the difficult choice.

Similar recommendations have emerged from nearly all the consensus conferences on screening. For example, Winawer and colleagues [11] reviewed the literature on screening for colon and rectal cancer. They did find evidence suggesting that screening provides a small benefit for men and women older than 50 years of age. However, their review of the evidence did not support any specific approach to screening. They considered flexible sigmoidoscopy, fecal occult blood tests, colonoscopy, and barium enemas. Each of these approaches is associated with a profile of risks and benefits. Ultimately, the group recommended that the decision be made by an informed patient.

Another related example concerns screening for prostate cancer in older men. As noted earlier, prostate cancer is common among older men. Yet, most of those diagnosed with the disease will die of other causes before their first symptom of prostate cancer. On behalf of the American College of Physicians, Coley and colleagues concluded that decisions about screening should be shared between well-informed patients and their physicians [12].

The need for patient involvement is even more clear when providers are uncertain about the appropriate options. When patients are asked to comply with medical regimens, they assume that the doctor is certain or confident that the diagnosis is correct and the proposed treatment is the best one available. A traditional model assumes that diagnostic tests give definitive diagnostic information. However, most medical decisions involve a fair degree of uncertainty. Furthermore, physicians do not use information in a systematic way. In one detailed analysis, Moskowitz, Kuipers, and Kassirer [13] analyzed how practicing physicians made difficult clinical decisions by studying transcripts of the doctors "thinking out loud." When these decisions were compared to results from systematic quantitative decision analysis, they found that clinicians made systematic errors in the use of information. Furthermore, there is substantial variability in conclusions reached by different physicians after examining the same clinical cases [14].

Why Shared Decisions are Necessary

Medical sciences are imprecise. Treatments typically have profiles of benefits and consequences. Patients may elect to use treatments if they perceive that the benefits outweigh the consequences. Several studies have shown how patient participation may improve medical outcomes [15]. For example, Greenfield, Kaplan, and Ware [16] randomly assigned patients with peptic ulcer disease to either be taught how to extract information from their provider or to receive didactic information about peptic ulcers. Those given brief training had more positive interactions with their physicians and later had better health, as measured by their ability to perform their usual activities. A similar study for patients with diabetes showed that those who are trained to actively participate in decisions about their care had significantly better control of their diabetes than those randomly assigned simply to receive standard information about diabetes [17].

Perhaps the most interesting set of findings demonstrates that patients who actively choose a treatment may obtain better outcomes than those assigned to a treatment by someone else. Experimental studies consistently support "direct effects" of compliance, which means that compliant patients do better, regardless of what they comply with [18]. Epstein reviewed six experimental studies in different areas of behavior intervention and medical care. In each of these studies, patients who complied with treatment had better health outcomes than those who did not. However, the effects were consistently found for placebo as well as for active treatment. In other words, the act of deciding to stay with a program results in better health outcomes. This effect may be as important as the nature of the medication itself. Choice and commitment to treatment may be a crucial component of treatment efficacy.

Often, patients come to treatment expecting benefit. However, experienced clinicians are aware that not all patients benefit from each episode of treatment, even under apparently identical circumstances. Most health outcomes are probabilistic [19]. To complicate matters even more, most patients expect their physicians to make a perfectly reliable diagnosis for each of their medical problems, but perfection in diagnosis could happen only in an ideal world: A patient could approach a physician with a list of symptoms and problems. Then the physician would identify the problem and administer a remedy that cured the ailment. The service would be inexpensive, effective, and painless. However, a substantial literature suggests that medical decisions rarely meet these ideals [20].

As mentioned earlier, the emerging healthcare paradigm of shared decision-making is a process in which patients and physicians join in a partnership to evaluate the alternatives for a particular medical decision [1, 21, 22, 23]. Patients and physicians have multiple options when confronted with most medical problems. In shared decision-making, the dyad begins with the recognition that there is uncertainty about diagnostic and treatment pathways for many conditions. Patients learn of the risks and benefits associated with each option and often participate in guided exercises to help them understand the consequences of different alternatives. Information can be presented using a variety of formats [24]. Many components of healthcare decisions involve factors that cannot be known by the healthcare provider. For example, many decisions involve concerns about sexual side effects or the effects of surgery on physical appearance. Shared decision-making involves elicitation of these preferences and their integration into the formal decision process.

The Reliability and Consistency of Clinical Decisions

The traditional biomedical model treats disease as a binary variable. People are sick or they are not. However, most chronic diseases are gradual processes and cannot be classified as binary. The threshold for deciding whether someone has the disease can be ambiguous, and as we have seen it may shift over time, with changing attitudes and technologies. Chapters 6–8 demonstrated that biological variables, such as cholesterol levels, blood pressure, and blood glucose, are normally distributed in the population. For most of these variables, an expert panel decides that a certain point along the continuum separates disease from nondisease. For several conditions, variable values now considered risk factors for disease were considered completely normal only a few years ago [25]. Within the past few years, lower diagnostics thresholds have been set for blood pressure [26], blood glucose [27], and cholesterol [28]. Setting diagnostic thresholds has a substantial impact upon healthcare costs. Pharmaceutical companies, for example, benefit significantly from lowered diagnostic thresholds because each time the threshold is lowered, a significantly larger portion of the population is eligible to use particular drugs.

Compounding the uncertainties in the new definitions of disease is the variability of judgments made in the interpretation of clinical data. Using both their experience and their knowledge of new standards, clinicians examine and interpret clinical information and make judgments about patients' conditions. Like any judgments, these are not always reliable. It is a well-known fact that physicians are highly variable in their interpretation of clinical data. They disagree with one another when examining the same clinical information [29]. And they disagree with themselves when presented with the same information at two points in time. Many examples support this claim. For instance, one study gave cardiologists high-quality angiograms and asked them to say if the stenosis in the left anterior descending artery was greater than 50 percent. This judgment is important because it is usually the threshold for revascularization of the coronary arteries. The study showed that the clinicians disagreed with one another in about 60 percent of the cases [30]. In another study, cardiologists were given the same angiograms at two different times. At the second assessment, they disagreed with their own first judgment in 8 percent to 37 percent of the cases [31].

Another study evaluated the reliability of pathologists'—assessments of ductile carcinoma in situ (DCIS). Six experienced pathologists were given written guidelines and examples of each of the problems for which they were looking. Following this training, they were given 24 high-quality slides of breast tissue. There was considerable variability in the propensity to see DCIS. One pathologist saw cancer in 12 percent of the slides while another saw DCIS in 33 percent of the same slides. Among 10 slides where at least one pathologist saw DCIS, no two pathologists had the same pattern of identification. One case was diagnosed by only one pathologist, and only two cases were seen by all six

[32, 33]. These variations in diagnostic patterns imply that patients with the same problem, going to different doctors, may get different diagnoses.

Do Patients Want to Participate in Decision-Making?

It is often argued that patients do not want to become involved in the decision process. Frequently, physicians remark that their patients want decisions made for them. There is now a substantial body of evidence that addresses this topic. Even the earliest studies on cancer patients found that the majority (62.5 percent) wanted to be involved in clinical decisions [34]. Younger patients are more interested in participating in clinical decisions than are older patients [35]. Among cancer patients, at least two-thirds prefer some level of collaboration in the process [36].

It is true, however, that not all studies suggest that patients want to be involved in the decision-making process. Interest in involvement is clearly associated not only with being younger [37], as just noted, but also with having higher levels of education [38]. Some evidence suggests that patients who are more seriously ill may also be willing to give their physicians a larger role in decision-making [39].

One of the important problems is that some patients seem to be unaware that there are alternatives [1, 40]. As noted in Chapters 5–8, most patients today are presented with a steady flow of information indicating that treatment is likely a very good idea for most medical problems. An interesting study by Dobias [41] analyzed the content of messages about mammography in popular magazines. The study found that magazines targeted at women with less education presented one-sided arguments urging the use of mammography. Magazines with a readership of more highly educated women tended to present both sides of the argument, but still slanted the message toward getting the test.

What Is the Patient's Role in Making Decisions?

Patients are getting more involved in decision-making, and this seems to be happening for several reasons. First, there is an increase in patient autonomy. The healthcare system is gradually coming to recognize that patients have an important independent role in the decision process. Second, the Internet has provided much greater access to health information. Third, clinicians now have many more options to offer patients. Fourth, healthcare costs are rising and not all choices are affordable. Fifth, many more people are experiencing chronic illness, and as a result, self-management is becoming an important consideration for those requiring long-term healthcare. Sixth, trade-offs are becoming more complicated; patients must consider both the risks and the benefits of treatment and understanding or at least have a feel for the complex probabilities involved. Seventh and last, there is a growing recognition that patients' personal values and rights are important and must be factored into the decision process [42].

In order to have true shared decision-making, the patient must have a clear understanding of the risks associated with his or her medical condition. A patient with high blood pressure, for example, must understand the increased risk of stroke and heart attack. This information should be presented as both absolute risk and relative risk. The patient must also have a clear understanding of the options available. The risk and benefits of each alternative treatment should be made available in a format that can be easily comprehended. Patents should also go through exercises that allow them to value the potential benefits and harms of the alternative treatments. For example, surgery for prostate cancer can make a man incontinent or impotent. For some men impotence might be a great concern, while other men are not sexually active and fear impotence less. Assessment of these values is an important component of shared decision-making. Finally, shared decision-making requires active participation in the decision process. Both patient and provider must be involved players in the process.

Shared decision-making is challenging for both patients and providers. Clinicians close their ears because they are busy and find it difficult to review all the options. On the other hand, informing patients about the risks and the benefits of the different alternatives may significantly reduce the chances that the doctor will be sued.

Shared decision-making also tends to take advantage of new sources of information, especially by patients, with all the attendant benefits and pitfalls. This is most obvious in the case of the Internet. Not only do patients now routinely find information on their medical problems on websites, they are just as often as not overwhelmed with information, and the quality and objectivity of the available material is often open to question. Leaving aside the obvious quacks and charlatans, patients also encounter impressive presentations of information that subtly or not subtly advocate a certain procedure, institution, or product. Figure 10.1, for example, shows a web page promoting LIPITOR. This impressive site offers patients a very positive slant on the value of the medication without the required balancing concerns noted in the company's own literature. It also describes the benefits in terms of relative risk gains rather than absolute risk changes. After reading this information, patients are likely to feel that there are many benefits and few risks of this medication.

Besides corporate- or sponsor-driven websites, there are now also internet-based decision aids that go a long way in helping patients develop an objective appraisal of medical information. These aids, which are becoming increasingly popular, include product publications, decision boards, videos, and audio-guided workbooks. Well-designed decision aids can coach patients through some of the difficult alternatives. The Cochran Collaborative, for example, now provides an inventory of patient decision aids and has over 50 web-based tools. These can be accessed at decisionaid.ohri.ca/AZinvent.php

Important information about LIPITOR

In September 2005, the U.S. Food and Drug Administration (FDA) approved the cholesterol-lowering therapy LIPITOR®
(atorvastatin calcium) for reducing the risk of stroke and heart attack in people with type 2 diabetes, near normal
cholesterol, and at least one other risk factor, such as high blood pressure or smoking. LIPITOR also received approval to
reduce the risk of stroke in people without evidence of heart disease but with multiple risk factors other than diabetes.

The FDA's decision pertaining to type 2 diabetes was based on the findings of the Collaborative Atorvastatin Diabetes
Study (CARDS). CARDS was a landmark trial of more than 2,800 patients with type 2 diabetes who had near normal
cholesterol but at least one other risk factor for heart attack.

The CARDS study showed that patients on LIPITOR experienced nearly 50 percent fewer strokes than those on
placebo. The trial was stopped nearly 2 years earlier than planned by the study's Steering Committee because of the
strong benefits among patients who took LIPITOR.

The additional approval of LIPITOR to reduce the risk of stroke in patients with multiple risk factors not including diabetes
reflects findings from the Anglo-Scandinavian Cardiac Outcomes Trial: Lipid-Lowering Arm (ASCOT-LLA). This study was
also halted nearly 2 years earlier than planned after it was found that LIPITOR reduced the relative risk of stroke by 26
percent compared with placebo.

The ASCOT-LLA study involved more than 10,300 people with normal or borderline cholesterol and no prior history of
heart disease, but with controlled high blood pressure and at least 3 other risk factors for heart disease, such as family
history, age over 55, smoking, diabetes and obesity.

"Patients with multiple risk factors, including diabetes, face a greater threat of heart attack and stroke, so reducing their
risk is critical," said David Waters, M.D., F.A.C.C., Chief of Cardiology, San Francisco General Hospital, San Francisco,
CA. "The idea that we can reduce the risk of heart attack and stroke even in this high-risk population with a drug like
LIPITOR is important."

CVD Impact

Every year, more than 865,000 Americans suffer a heart attack. There are 7.8 million people in the United States who are
heart attack survivors. High blood pressure and elevated cholesterol are leading risk factors for heart disease but other
factors compound the risk, including family history of heart disease, age, smoking, diabetes, obesity and lack of exercise.
Direct (medical costs) and indirect (lost productivity) costs related to coronary heart disease are expected to exceed$133
billion in 2004.[1]

LIPITOR is the most prescribed cholesterol-lowering therapy in the world with more than 100 million patient years of
experience. Since the introduction of LIPITOR 7 years ago, its safety and effectiveness have been supported through the
Atorvastatin Landmark Program™, an extensive clinical program with more than 400 ongoing and completed trials
involving more than 80,000 patients.

Fig. 10.1 Advertisement for LIPITOR aimed at direct marketing to patients. From: http://www.lipitor.com/cwp/appmanager/lipitor/lipitorDesktop?_nfpb=true&_pageLabel=ascotLLA

Ultimately, of course, the goal is to send patients to a legitimate website where they interact with decision tools, then provide an opportunity to discuss the alternatives with a compassionate healthcare provider.

Shared Decision-Making and the Overuse of Medical Services

When presented with the full picture of information about the risks and benefits of treatments, patients often make conservative choices, as demonstrated in the three following examples. The first involves back surgery.

Back pain is the leading cause of visits to orthopedic surgeons and neuro-surgeons in the USA, and the USA has a significantly higher rate of back surgery than any other developed country [43, 44]. However, these surgeries are not always necessary, and in most cases, the surgery is elective and there is reason to believe that medication alone may produce equivalent results [45]. A recent clinical trial compared surgery versus prolonged conservative treatment for adults with radiologist confirmed herniated disks. The surgery patients received surgical treatment within two weeks while the other group got physical therapy and medical support. Some of these patients eventually chose to have surgery. Although the surgery patients got better sooner, after 1 year, the outcomes for the two groups were equivalent [46]. Richard Deyo reviewed a series of surgical trials and considered the question, "who needs back surgery." Clearly, surgery is necessary for those who have major motor deficits because of disk problems and those who have had trauma to the spine. Most people with herniated disks or spinal stenosis, according to Deyo, do not need surgery. Surgery may offer pain relief, but that comes with some risks. For most patients, shared decision-making is the recommended method for finding the best pathway [47].

Deyo and his colleagues conducted a systematic clinical trial to evaluate the choices back-surgery patients made after an opportunity for shared decision-making. The patients participated at either the Group Health Cooperative in Seattle, Washington, or at the University of Iowa. The 393 patients who were candidates for elective back surgery were randomly assigned to an interactive video explaining the risks and benefits of back surgery or to a control group. (Both groups got a booklet describing back surgery.) The patients had either a herniated disk, spinal stenosis, or other related diagnoses. The outcome was cumulative probability that the patients received surgery at some point after they had been randomly assigned to a treatment condition. The time variable is represented as days following randomization on the x-axis of the graph. Patients who watched the interactive video were significantly less likely to have surgery than those in the control group (see Fig. 10.2). The difference was most apparent for patients with herniated discs, who may have been the least likely to benefit from surgery. Patients with spinal stenosis were slightly more likely to have surgery after they had watched the video, but the difference was not statistically significant. Surgery is believed to be a better clinical option for these patients because outcomes are often favorable.

Although there were few differences observed in patient satisfaction, the patients in the video group felt better informed. Symptoms and functional outcomes were measured 3 months and 1 year after the patients had been assigned to the conditions. The differences were not statistically significant. Overall, the study demonstrated that exposure to balanced information reduces the number of back surgeries without any adverse consequences on health outcome [48]. The reduction was most likely in the clinical group that was least likely to benefit from surgery.

The second example comes from a study on the use of adjuvant breast cancer treatment. Women with breast cancer are confronted with a very difficult series of choices, and these choices have been made all the more complex by recent

Fig. 10.2 Cumulative probability of surgery as a function of time from being randomly assigned to a video disk for shared decision-making (plus a booklet) or to a booklet-only condition. (From Deyo et al. [48].)

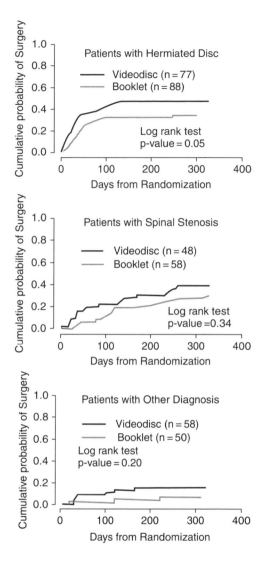

changes in treatment guidelines. Until very recently, most women with early-stage breast cancer were advised to get adjuvant chemotherapy. A variety of newer findings, however, have raised questions about the blanket recommendation for these therapies. First, newer medications, known as Aromatase Inhibitors, may offer better outcomes for some women because they produce fewer side effects than do traditional chemotherapies. But the most important change in guidelines concerns age. Following menopause, many women have breast cancer that is estrogen-receptor positive. This means the women have tumors that are sensitive to estrogen. In contrast, women before menopause are more likely to have estrogen-receptor negative breast cancer. These women may have tumors that are less affected by estrogen. For older women with estrogen-receptor positive breast cancer, chemotherapy may offer few benefits. The most recent change in guidelines now suggests a careful evaluation of the use of adjuvant chemotherapy. Thus, the choice of therapy for women with low tumor severity has become a more difficult decision.

One study noted that oncologists were highly variable in the information they provide to breast-cancer patients. Many provide no information and simply place all women on adjuvant therapy. A study by Pamela Peele and colleagues randomly assigned 386 women with breast cancer to either an information pamphlet about adjuvant therapy or an evidence-based decision aid. The study showed a significant reduction in the choice to get adjuvant chemotherapy among the women who had used the decision aid; in this group, 35 of 60 women (58 percent) chose adjuvant therapy. In contrast, the rate of those who chose to use adjuvant therapy was 87 percent (33 of 38 women) in the "usual-care" control group (see Fig. 10.3).

The most recent evidence suggests that women with low tumor severity have relatively little to gain from intensive adjuvant chemotherapy. However, the chemotherapy causes significant side effects. The use of decision aids appeared to significantly reduce the number of women who chose this option. The same study found fewer differences between women with medium tumor severity or higher tumor severity. In fact, among women with high tumor severity, for which adjuvant therapy was less controversial, women using the decision aid were slightly (although not statistically significantly) more likely to select adjuvant therapy [49].

The third example comes from a study on screening for prostate cancer. Frosch, Kaplan, and Feletti [50] considered a decision aid to help men decide whether they should be screened for prostate cancer using the PSA test. The men were all enrolled in a clinic that provides a wide variety of medical screening tests. In an experiment, the men were assigned to one of four groups that form the cells of a matrix. One factor was for use of a decision video. Men either

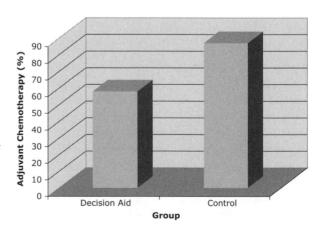

Fig. 10.3 The percentage of women choosing adjuvant chemotherapy with and without decision aids. (Adapted from Peele et al. [49].)

watched or did not watch a video that systematically reviewed the risks and benefits of PSA screening. The video featured a debate between a urologist who favored PSA screening and an internist who opposed PSA screening. Furthermore, the video systematically reviewed the probabilities of false positives, false negatives, and the risks of prostate cancer. It also systematically reviewed the evidence for the benefits of treatment for prostate cancer. The other factor in the experimental design was whether men had the opportunity to discuss the decision with others. The experimental design thus resulted in the creation of four groups: usual care, discussion alone, video alone, and video plus discussion. All men were asked if they wanted the PSA test, and medical records were obtained to determine whether the test was completed.

The study showed that there was a systematic effect of the video and discussion groups. In the usual-care control group, virtually all men (97 percent) got the PSA test. In other words, with no new information, men will typically take the test. In the other groups, having more information led to a conservative bias. In contrast to the usual-care control, those in the other groups were more sensitive to the risks of the test in relation to its benefits. Among those participating in the discussion group, 82 percent got the PSA test. For those watching the video, 63 percent completed the test. Those watching the video and participating in the discussions had only a 50-percent PSA completion rate (see Fig. 10.4). The study demonstrates that, as patients become better informed, they are less likely to take the PSA test. The study also obtained information on patient knowledge about the PSA test and prostate cancer. As knowledge increased, the likelihood of getting the PSA test decreased, again, stressing that better-informed patients make more conservative decisions.

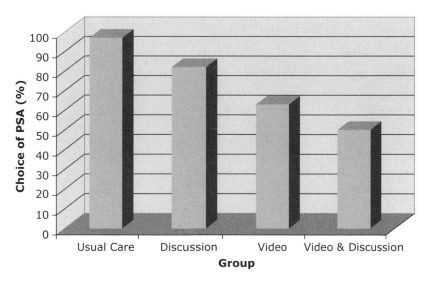

Fig. 10.4 Percentage of men choosing PSA after information interventions. (Adapted from Frosch et al. [50].)

As mentioned earlier, the Internet has significant advantages as a tool for implementing shared decision-making. Medical knowledge changes very quickly, so the Internet, with its unique ability to present updated information, is an ideal medium for publishing the latest medical findings and trends. However, we do not know how effective the Internet is at actually delivering information. New evidence suggests that large proportions of the general population have Internet access. Yet, how well does the Internet deliver information in a way that enables shared decision-making?

In one study, 226 men, 50 years of age or older, who are scheduled for a complete physical exam, were randomly assigned to access a website or to view a 23-minute videotape about the risks and benefits of being screened for prostate cancer using the PSA test. Both methods of delivering the information were effective, but those watching the video were more likely to review the materials than those watching on the Internet. In addition, those watching the video were more likely to increase their knowledge about the PSA test and were more likely to decline the test than those assigned to the Internet group. Furthermore, those who watched the video were more likely to express confidence that watchful waiting was the best treatment for prostate cancer. Thus, it appeared that the video may have been the best channel for delivering the information. However, using cookies from the Internet, it was possible to determine how much time each participant spent using the program. The analysis indicated that many of the men spent very little time with the Internet program. Among those men who participated in the entire Internet program, the results were identical to those who watched the video. In other words, the Internet and the video worked about equally as well if people exposed themselves to the entire program. When motivated and technologically equipped to use the Internet, patients can gain significant benefits [51].

Consumer-Driven Health Plans

When consumers get involved in healthcare decisions, they typically make good choices. A relatively new approach to health insurance offers patients more opportunities to allocate their own healthcare resources. A good plan gives the patient an account and allows him or her to spend on basic services and prescriptions. The plans have a safety component that covers patients in the event of serious disease or large expenses. Information services give patients balanced information for shared decision-making. One industry-sponsored study evaluated more than 1,000 participants in consumer-directed plans in comparison with about 2,500 patients in traditional plans. Those in consumer-driven plans were 25 percent more likely to engage in healthy behaviors, 30 percent more likely to get annual check ups, 20 percent more likely to engage in good self-care for their chronic conditions, and 50 percent more likely to ask about costs. Overall, the participants in these plans spent less on care and engaged in behaviors that would improve their own health while making themselves less dependent on the healthcare system [52].

Conclusions

Decisions about healthcare can be very difficult. It is common for evidence supporting treatment to be ambiguous or for decisions to require trade-offs between side effects and benefits of treatment. Components of the decision might be very personal, like whether a man is willing to risk impotence or whether a woman is willing to lose a significant portion of her breast.

Until recently, physicians felt empowered to make the best decisions for their patients. However, times are changing, and quality standards now emphasize the consideration of patient preferences. A variety of methods and decision aids are now available to help patients address choices when the evidence is conflicted or ambiguous.

Studies on shared medical decision-making tend to show that patients want to be involved in the process and that they often make conservative decisions. Shared decision-making is a true exercise in informed consent, and it may help providers avoid lawsuits. Thus, shared decision-making may lead to fewer unnecessary tests and interventions and to lower healthcare costs.

References

1. Frosch DL, Kaplan RM. Shared decision making in clinical medicine: past research and future directions. *Am J Prev Med.* 1999;17(4):285–294.
2. Kaplan RM, Frosch DL. Decision making in medicine and health care. *Annu Rev Clin Psychol.* 2005;1:525–556.
3. Russell LB, Milbank Memorial Fund. *Educated Guesses: Making Policy about Medical Screening Tests.* Berkeley, CA: University of California Press; 1994.
4. Kaplan RM, Navarro A. Mammography screening: prospects and opportunity costs. *Women's Health: Research on Gender, Behavioral, and Policy.* 1996;2(209–233.):209–233.
5. Fletcher SW. Breast cancer screening among women in their forties: an overview of the issues. *J Natl Cancer Inst Monogr.* 1997;(22):5–9.
6. Fletcher SW. Whither scientific deliberation in health policy recommendations? Alice in the Wonderland of breast-cancer screening. *N Engl J Med.* Apr 17 1997;336(16):1180–1183.
7. Eddy DM. Screening for breast cancer. *Ann Intern Med.* Sep 1 1989;111(5):389–399.
8. Elmore JG, Barton MB, Moceri VM, Polk S, Arena PJ, Fletcher SW. Ten-year risk of false positive screening mammograms and clinical breast examinations. *New Engl J Med.* Apr 16 1998;338(16):1089–1096.
9. Porzsolt F, Leonhardt-Huober H, Kaplan RM. Aims and value of screening: Is perceived safety a value for which to pay? In F. Porzsolt & RM Kaplan (Eds). Optimizing Health: Improving the value of healthcare delivery. New York: Springer, 2006, pgs 199–204.
10. Roberts R, Bell H, Wall E, Moy J, Hess G, Bower H. Trial of labor or repeated cesarean section: the woman's choice. *Arch Fam Med.* 1997;6(2):120–125.

11. Winawer SJ, Fletcher RH, Miller L, et al. Colorectal cancer screening: clinical guidelines and rationale. *Gastroenterology*. Feb 1997;112(2):594–642.
12. Coley CM, Barry MJ, Fleming C, Fahs MC, Mulley AG. Early detection of prostate cancer. Part II: Estimating the risks, benefits, and costs. American College of Physicians [see comments]. *Ann Inter Med*. 1997;126(6):468–479.
13. Moskowitz AJ, Kuipers BJ, Kassirer JP. Dealing with uncertainty, risks, and tradeoffs in clinical decisions: a cognitive science approach. *Ann Intern Med*. Mar 1988;108(3): 435–449.
14. Burnand B, Feinstein AR. The role of diagnostic inconsistency in changing rates of occurrence for coronary heart disease. *J Clin Epidemiol*. Sep 1992;45(9):929–940.
15. Kaplan SH, Greenfield S, Ware JE, Jr. Assessing the effects of physician-patient interactions on the outcomes of chronic disease. *Med Care*. Mar 1989;27(3 Suppl):S110–S127.
16. Greenfield S, Kaplan S, Ware JE, Jr. Expanding patient involvement in care: effects on patient outcomes. *Ann Intern Med*. 1985;102(4):520–528.
17. Greenfield S, Kaplan SH, Ware JE, Jr., Yano EM, Frank HJ. Patients' participation in medical care: effects on blood sugar control and quality of life in diabetes. *J Gen Intern Med*. Sep–Oct 1988;3(5):448–457.
18. Epstein LH. The direct effects of compliance on health outcome. *Health Psychol*. 1984;3(4):385–393.
19. Ratliff A, Angell M, Dow RW, et al. What is a good decision? *Eff Clin Pract*. Jul–Aug 1999;2(4):185–197.
20. Eddy DM. Clinical decision making: from theory to practice. Designing a practice policy. Standards, guidelines, and options. *JAMA*. Jun 13 1990;263(22):3077, 3081, 3084.
21. Elwyn G, Edwards A, Gwyn R, Grol R. Towards a feasible model for shared decision making: focus group study with general practice registrars. [comment]. *BMJ*. 1999; 319(7212):753–756.
22. Wolf AM, Schorling JB. Does informed consent alter elderly patients' preferences for colorectal cancer screening? Results of a randomized trial. *J Gen Intern Med*. Jan 2000;15(1):24–30.
23. Woolf SH. Shared decision-making: the case for letting patients decide which choice is best. [comment]. *J Fam Pract*. 1997;45(3):205–208.
24. O'Connor AM, Stacey D, Entwistle V, et al. Decision aids for people facing health treatment or screening decisions. *Cochrane Database Syst Rev*. 2003;(2):CD001431.
25. Kaplan RM. Effects of changes in diagnostic thresholds on healthcare for older adults. In: Aldwin CM, Spiro AI, Park C, eds. *Handbook of the Health Psychology and Aging*. New York: Guilford Press; 2006.
26. Chobanian AV, Bakris GL, Black HR, et al. Seventh Report of the Joint National Committee on Prevention, Detection, Evaluation, and Treatment of High Blood Pressure. *Hypertension*. Dec 2003;42(6):1206–1252.
27. Genuth S, Alberti KG, Bennett P, et al. Follow-up report on the diagnosis of diabetes mellitus. *Diabetes Care*. Nov 2003;26(11):3160–3167.
28. Grundy SM, Cleeman JI, Merz CN, et al. Implications of recent clinical trials for the National Cholesterol Education Program Adult Treatment Panel III guidelines. *Circulation*. Jul 13 2004;110(2):227–239.
29. Eddy DM. Evidence-based medicine: a unified approach. *Health Aff (Millwood)*. Jan–Feb 2005;24(1):9–17.
30. Zir LM, Miller SW, Dinsmore RE, Gilbert JP, Harthorne JW. Interobserver variability in coronary angiography. *Circulation*. 1976;53(4):627–632.
31. Detre KM, Wright E, Murphy ML, Takaro T. Observer agreement in evaluating coronary angiograms. *Circulation*. 1975;52(6):979–986.
32. Schnitt SJ, Connolly JL, Tavassoli FA, et al. Interobserver reproducibility in the diagnosis of ductal proliferative breast lesions using standardized criteria [see comments]. *Am J Surg Pathol*. 1992;16(12):1133–1143.

33. Welch HG. *Should I be Tested for Cancer?* Berkeley, CA: University of California Press; 2004.
34. Cassileth BR, Zupkis RV, Sutton-Smith K, March V. Information and participation preferences among cancer patients. *Ann Intern Med.* 1980;92(6):832–836.
35. Blanchard CG, Labrecque MS, Ruckdeschel JC, Blanchard EB. Information and decision-making preferences of hospitalized adult cancer patients. *Soc Sci Med.* 1988;27(11): 1139–1145.
36. Degner LF, Sloan JA, Venkatesh P. The control preferences scale. *Can J Nurs Res.* Fall 1997;29(3):21–43.
37. Arora NK, McHorney CA. Patient preferences for medical decision making: who really wants to participate? *Med Care.* Mar 2000;38(3):335–341.
38. Krupat E, Bell RA, Kravitz RL, Thom D, Azari R. When physicians and patients think alike: patient-centered beliefs and their impact on satisfaction and trust. *J Fam Pract.* Dec 2001;50(12):1057–1062.
39. Rosen P, Anell A, Hjortsberg C. Patient views on choice and participation in primary health care. *Health Policy.* Feb 2001;55(2):121–128.
40. Sepucha KR, Mulley AG. Extending decision support: preparation and implementation. *Patient Educ Couns.* Jul 2003;50(3):269–271.
41. Dobias KS, Moyer CA, McAchran SE, Katz SJ, Sonnad SS. Mammography messages in popular media: implications for patient expectations and shared clinical decision-making. *Health Expect.* 2001;4(2):127–135.
42. Woolf SH, Chan EC, Harris R, et al. Promoting informed choice: transforming health care to dispense knowledge for decision making. *Ann Intern Med.* Aug 16 2005;143(4): 293–300.
43. Deyo RA, Gray DT, Kreuter W, Mirza S, Martin BI. United States trends in lumbar fusion surgery for degenerative conditions. *Spine.* Jun 15 2005;30(12):1441–1445; discussion 1446–1447.
44. Deyo RA, Mirza SK. Trends and variations in the use of spine surgery. *Clin Orthop Relat Res.* Feb 2006;443:139–146.
45. Saal JA, Saal JS. Nonoperative treatment of herniated lumbar intervertebral disc with radiculopathy: an outcome study. *Spine.* Apr 1989;14(4):431–437.
46. Peul WC, van Houwelingen HC, van den Hout WB, et al. Surgery versus prolonged conservative treatment for sciatica. *N Engl J Med.* May 31 2007;356(22):2245–2256.
47. Deyo RA. Back surgery – who needs it? *N Engl J Med.* May 31 2007;356(22):2239–2243.
48. Deyo RA, Cherkin DC, Weinstein J, Howe J, Ciol M, Mulley AG, Jr. Involving patients in clinical decisions: impact of an interactive video program on use of back surgery. *Med Care.* Sep 2000;38(9):959–969.
49. Peele PB, Siminoff LA, Xu Y, Ravdin PM. Decreased use of adjuvant breast cancer therapy in a randomized controlled trial of a decision aid with individualized risk information. *Med Decis Making.* May–Jun 2005;25(3):301–307.
50. Frosch DL, Kaplan RM, Felitti V. The evaluation of two methods to facilitate shared decision making for men considering the prostate-specific antigen test. *J Gen Intern Med.* Jun 2001;16(6):391–398.
51. Frosch DL, Kaplan RM, Felitti VJ. A randomized controlled trial comparing internet and video to facilitate patient education for men considering the prostate specific antigen test. *J Gen Intern Med.* Oct 2003;18(10):781–787.
52. McKinsey & Company. *Consumer-Directed Health Plan Report – Early Evidence is Promising* 2005.

Chapter 11
Putting the Pieces Together

This book has addressed a variety of important medical and healthcare topics. On the surface, the topics may not have been obviously connected to one another. This final chapter suggests how the pieces of the puzzle fit together.

Costs are Out of Control

Healthcare is the largest sector in the economies of most developed countries [1]. We have been unable to control healthcare costs. US healthcare costs grew from 4 percent of the gross domestic product in the 1960 s to nearly 15 percent today [2]. In addition, the increase in healthcare costs contributes to increases in prices for products manufactured by companies that provide health benefits for their employees. General Motors, for example, until recently the world's largest automobile producer, is currently on the verge of bankruptcy in large part because it has been unable to control expenses. And one of the largest expenses it has failed to control is its health-insurance cost for employees and retirees. Many American industries are attempting to restructure in order to get out from under healthcare costs. For workers, it is a losing battle. Take California workers as an example. Their premium contributions for single coverage had increased 127.9 percent between 2001 and 2006. During that same interval, their cumulative earnings increased cumulatively by 11.9 percent.

For obvious reasons, subsidized or "free" healthcare services are attractive to individuals, who reasonably want the best possible medical services at the lowest possible cost. Who would not want a life made healthier, happier, and longer thanks to the benefits of the very best modern medicine? Healthcare services are also attractive to corporations and other employers—to recruit and retain talented hardworking people, to improve the overall health and therefore the productivity of their workforce, and to enhance their image as enlightened, humane institutions. However, as well articulated by Ezekiel Emanuel and Victor Fuchs, the belief that someone else is paying for our healthcare is a myth [3]. Employers do not really pay for healthcare because these costs are passed on to households through lower wages and higher consumer prices.

R.M. Kaplan, *Disease, Diagnoses, and Dollars*, DOI 10.1007/978-0-387-74045-4_11,   167
© Springer Science+Business Media, LLC 2009

When government pays for healthcare, it does it through higher taxes, or greater borrowing. In the end, there is no free lunch (or healthcare). The cost is borne by ordinary citizens.

There is the proverbial elephant sitting in the room, and though we all know it, we find it hard even to acknowledge: Healthcare costs are out of control, and in order to begin to control them, we will have to make tough decisions about what services are necessary and what services provide best value for patients.

The Proliferation of Services

The problem is beyond services costing too much: It is also that there are too many services being offered and used—including many with little value. This is partly due to improvements in diagnostic technology that have led to significant increases in the rate of disease identified within communities. Several chapters in this book discuss the problem of pseudodisease. This is disease which, although identifiable, will not have adverse effects on untreated patients. In the future, we will be challenged to select not only treatments but also diagnostic tests. Patients diagnosed with a disease are likely to demand treatment, and qualify for insurance coverage of their treatment, even when the value of treatment is expected to be low. Pseudodisease deserves attention because it is the diagnostic gateway to ineffective, and sometimes potentially harmful, treatment.

One way to think about our problem is that making money in medicine and healthcare is dependent on the size of the market. The market size of very sick people is quiet small. The market is bigger when we consider people who are mildly ill. The best way to make the market big enough for large profits is to make well people sick. Essentially, that is what has been accomplished with the new definitions of disease.

In the simplest terms, I have argued that the key to our healthcare crisis is volume: too much diagnosis, too much treatment, and too much medication. The solution does require health insurance for all people, but not to provide *all* services for *all* people. The first half of the sentence is easy to swallow, but the second half is harder to take. We all want the best care for ourselves and for our families and nobody wants to second-guess their doctor. It is particularly disturbing that a doctor's advice would be ignored because some third party does not want to pay the bill. The Michael Moore documentary "Sicko" offered a series of horror stories resulting from denial of medical services by insurance companies. I imagine that many readers, even those who accept the premise that there is too much medical care, will have an adverse reaction to someone else deciding who will get more and who will get less medical care.

There is an uncomfortable tension over the control of healthcare and we need to face it head on. First, we need to address the argument that new medications produce little harm. In general, most of the new medications are well tolerated.

However, there are problems with almost any medication. The drugs have powerful effects, and it is rare to find a medication that does exactly one thing. It has been argued that the effects of cholesterol-lowering in the elderly are not well documented but that the chances of adverse drug reactions increase with age [4]. Over an extended period of use, we never know what unintended damage medicines will cause. Sometimes it takes years to discover the consequences of medication use. In the early 1970 s, lithium salts were believed to be the new magic bullet for the treatment of bipolar depression. Today, many of those patients treated with lithium are being treated for kidney failure caused by the medication [5]. When I was a child, my family doctor used antimicrobial drugs for nearly any illness. There was no downside he would argue. Today, the overuse of antimicrobial medications is credited with the re-emergence of tuberculosis and other infections that have evolved to be resistant to antibiotic therapies [6]. Just a few years ago, a new class of anti-inflammatory drugs, known as coxibs, was promoted as very effective and completely safe. Celebrex was the king of this class. However, a few years after introduction, evidence emerged documenting that celebrex increases the chances of death from heart disease [7]. Drugs are powerful biological agents. They often have effects that were unanticipated. When drugs are needed, it is worth taking the risk of side effects. But, is it worth taking the risk when there are few expected benefits?

A second concern is that the known consequences of treatment may be worse than the disease itself. The prostate cancer example has been discussed several times in the preceding chapters. For a man at great risk of losing his life to prostate cancer, trading longer life for impotence may be a wise choice. But, for many men, surgery is not believed to make life longer, and it is almost certain that it will make life less desirable [8].

The third concern is societal. Providing too much medicine for some insured people causes premiums to go up for everyone. This means that employers need to pay more and that can inflate the costs of products and services and make American products less competitive on world markets. It might also mean employees earn lower wages because more of the total compensation package goes to pay for benefits. Some employers may decide to cease their health insurance plans. When they do, more of their employees are left uncovered. Uninsured patients, when faced with emergencies, often fail to compensate doctors and hospitals for their care and these costs are passed along to the insured patients. The consequences of failing to control healthcare costs affect everyone.

You may have read this book as antimedical. There is no question that I have challenged the medical care system. But, I am a supporter of medicine. I have been a medical school professor for my entire adult life and I am not hesitant to go to doctors when I am sick. When needed, medicine extends lives and reduces suffering. The anitmedical tone addresses a different problem. When the use of medicines and medical care is unnecessary, it results in loss of money, causes anxiety, and may cause harm. The goal of this book was not to trash the medical care establishment. It was to encourage people to be better-informed consumers of medical care. By looking at the absolute risks and benefits of treatment and by engaging in shared medical decision-making, I believe patients will become better consumers for themselves of better stewards of our limited healthcare resources.

The one point on which there seems to be near consensus is that the American healthcare system is broken. Furthermore, the systems in other developed countries are beginning to face some of the problems that crippled the American system. Fixing these problems will be challenging, but there are some specific steps we can take to find our way out of the mess that now consumes us. Let us look at a few specific actions that might help.

Changes in Communications with Patients

We need to reconsider how patients get information. Several strategies should be considered, including:

- Patients need to become more involved in decision-making about their own care. The use of shared medical decision-making and decision aides should be expanded and programs such as Medicare and Medicaid should support these services.

The system may work better if informed patients are able to be more selfish—to look out for their own self-interests. Many people express qualms when they hear talk that emphasizes the role of self-interest in making choices. After all, selfishness sounds so ... selfish. Economists view selfishness differently. They believe it is required for economies to succeed. For example, individual decision-makers optimize their resources by choosing alternatives that give them the most satisfaction at the lowest cost. Markets work best if consumers attend to their own self-interest. When I shop to obtain the lowest price on a product, others will benefit because providers who want my business must offer the best service or product at the lowest cost. This competition will force the price of the product to be lower. Economists argue that selfishness—or "consumer sovereignty," to give it a more palatable name—is necessary and desirable.

Healthcare challenges many of these principles of self-interest and self-determination. Physicians and administrators have traditionally spoken for and made decisions on behalf of their patients. But things are changing. A growing literature suggests that patients are making more decisions independently of their healthcare providers. Patient preferences and prerogatives are beginning to find some acceptance among healthcare professionals, as they should. However, patients are often deprived of some of the information that they need to be really effective decision-makers. They are not able to purchase products that maximize the use of their own resources because many of the important products are controlled by prescription. Although most physicians want to act in the best interests of their patients, it is not clear that they fully understand patient preference when making these decisions. Tradeoffs, which are so important to economic thinking, are not valued in the same way by healthcare providers on one hand and their patients on the other.

Chapter 10 summarized a growing literature showing that patient decision aids are available and that they may have important effects on patient decisions. In particular, well-informed patients often opt out of unnecessary tests or procedures. The problem is that providers cannot be compensated for using these decision tools. To address this, we need to provide greater incentives for patient involvement in healthcare decisions. Medicare, for example, could create a provider payment code for use of a decision aid. Although they will spend more money for decision counseling, it is likely that there will be substantial savings through the reduction in the use of unneeded services. Research is needed to document these cost offsets.

There is, of course, a concern that those with a commercial interest in certain decisions will hijack decision aids. Pharmaceutical companies, for example, can be expected to create decision aids that direct patients toward their products. Like the FDA's impartial oversight over medicines, there may be a need for impartial supervision of evidence-based decision tools. However this evolves, I remain convinced that patients are motivated to protect both their own health and their own pocket books. With better information, they will make appropriate choices. We just need to offer them the right tools.

- Consumers should be given more information and more education on how to interpret risk information.

A lot of medical information is given to ill patients. Sometimes sorting out all this information can be very difficult. For example, one might be told that a medicine will make one better. But how likely is that benefit? Chapter 3 noted some of the discrepancies between the expectations people have of medicine and what is actually delivered. There are two problems. First, patients often think about disease using simple mechanical models of chronic illness, leading them to the incorrect assumption that there are simple mechanical cures. Fixing a narrowed coronary artery is much more complex than unplugging a clogged pipe. Second, popular media report benefits of healthcare in ways that may exaggerate expectations of benefit. For example, the benefits of a cholesterol-lowering medication might be promoted as reducing the chances of heart attack by 45 percent when the absolute change in risk for an individual patient may be less than 1 percent. It has been claimed that taking an aspirin every other day reduces the chance of a fatal heart attack by 72 percent. Evidence does suggest that the relative risk may decline by this amount. However, most patients are interested in how much their own individual risk changes. By taking aspirin every other day, evidence suggests that the chances of dying from a heart attack are reduced by approximately 0.1 percent (or about one-tenth of 1 percent) (see Chapter 3 page 28). A reduction of 0.1 percent is much less motivating than

72 percent. The inflated expectations of benefit may also result from promotional campaigns that play upon these misperceptions.

The different ways of reporting risks are confusing to both providers and patients, and it should be required that both absolute and relative risks be communicated to patients. Furthermore, we should be given information on the number of people who need to be treated to achieve one positive outcome (NNT) and the number of people treated before one case of harm occurs (NNH).

- Direct-to-consumer advertising should be restricted or eliminated. If it is continued, federal agencies should require balanced presentations of costs, risks, and benefits.

Much of the overuse of medication results from advertising campaigns that go directly to consumers. Advertising campaigns that deliberately mislead consumers are problematic. Direct-to-consumer advertising of pharmaceutical products is only allowed in two countries, the USA and New Zealand, and control over this "commercial speech" may be necessary. In the USA, direct-to-consumer advertising has run amuck. Direct-to-consumer advertising was not allowed in the USA until 1997. In the decade after it was introduced the number of advertisements grew exponentially [9]. Each year, American viewers may sit through up to 16 hours of paid advertisements guiding them to ask their doctors for specific trade-marked pharmaceutical products. These advertisements often stimulate consumers to request products that are not medically indicated, or more expensive than competing products with equivalent clinically efficacy.

The stated purpose of direct-to-consumer advertising is to inform patients about appropriate licensed products. The real purpose is to expand the markets for prescription medications. My UCLA colleague Dominick Frosch has done detailed studies of advertisement content and found that 95 percent of direct-to-consumer advertisements had strong emotional appeals. Although the advertisements are justified as mechanisms to educate patients, only about a quarter of them offer information about the disease, risk factors, or prevalence. A common theme in the advertisements is that diseases cause loss of control over some important aspect of life and that use of medication restores control. Even though most of the drugs advertised directly to consumers are modest variations on competing medications, 58 percent of the advertisements portray the promoted drug as a medical breakthrough. For many of the conditions, nondrug treatments such as diet and exercise, are recommended in treatment guidelines. None of the advertisements mentioned these alternatives, and only 19 percent acknowledged that nondrug approaches should be used along with drug treatment [10]. It is hard to justify direct-to-consumer advertising as a mechanism to inform patients because the information given to patients is incomplete and slanted. The real consequences are increased volume of medication use, increased costs, and greater financial pressure on the system.

There is ample justification for restricting direct-to-consumer advertising. All countries in the world, with the exception of the USA and New Zealand have such restrictions. Furthermore, the US system functioned quite adequately before accepting direct-to-consumer advertising in 1997. Under the US constitution, commercial speech is not given the same protection as free speech.

We Need to Re-examine the Process of Developing Practice Guidelines

Evidence-based medicine is an important new idea in healthcare. Evidence-based guidelines rely on systematic reviews of research studies to guide physicians in their medical decision-making. Increasingly, incentives have been used to get providers to comply with these guidelines. Some payers will only reimburse providers for services identified in guidelines. New approaches to pay for performance provide incentives for strict compliance to guidelines. However, the current process of guideline development leaves much to be desired.

In Chapters 5–8, we looked critically at the guidelines process. Although evidence-based guidelines are a good idea, it has also become clear that there are huge financial incentives for getting a service included in the guidelines. Although the guidelines are usually developed on the basis of peer consensus, it is not always clear that adherence to guidelines will result in patient benefit. Some cancer-screening tests appear to provide relatively little patient benefit (see Chapter 5). Furthermore, lowering of thresholds for high blood pressure (Chapter 6), high cholesterol (Chapter 7), or IFG (Chapter 8) may offer a small amount of benefit to some people, but are unlikely to benefit the great majority of people who are now classified as in need of regular medical care. The conclusion seems to be that there are few positive consequences of broadening the market for healthcare. But is this assumption correct? Evidence-based guidelines are on the right track, but they can be improved by a few policy changes, including:

• Evidence-based guidelines should consider both the probability and the possibility that a treatment will provide benefit.

It is naïve to think that extending the market for healthcare will not have important societal consequences. Let us begin with the development of guidelines. Guideline-development committees may think little harm is done by being more inclusive about who should be treated. However, under managed care, it will be very difficult to deny a service that has been identified as necessary by a guideline-development group, and it will be particularly difficult to deny a service when an expert panel feels this service mitigates a risk factor for serious disability or death. We know that most people who die of strokes do not have high blood pressure and that most people who die of heart disease do not have seriously elevated cholesterol. In the future, it is likely that doctors will be blamed if their untreated patients with relatively normal cholesterol or relatively normal blood pressure die of heart disease or stroke. For a variety of reasons, the impact of guidelines is likely to be a greatly expanded market for pharmaceutical products. This market expansion will lead to higher healthcare costs, but it is likely that population health benefits will be only minor.

To address this problem, the use of evidence-based patient guidelines needs to be rethought. There are several problems with current evidence-based guidelines. First, the definition of whether the treatment works can vary greatly. Different investigators measure different outcomes, and it is not always clear that the measures used in clinical studies are meaningful. A second problem is that guideline developers usually do not distinguish between the possibility and the probability that a patient will benefit. For example, it is possible that a patient with prehypertension will benefit from a medication that will lower blood pressure. However, the probability that he or she will benefit can be extremely low. According to our analysis, there is a minute possibility that a stroke can be avoided. At the same time, the probabilities that there will be increased cost and inconvenience are nearly certain. Newer guidelines are beginning to consider numbers needed to treat and numbers needed to harm. However, the expected impact on individual patients is rarely noted.

- An impartial government agency should be developed to oversee the guideline process.

Increased volume of drugs and medical services is big business. With so much money involved, there is substantial pressure to include specific services in practice guidelines. The Center for Responsible Politics reports on the amount of spending for healthcare lobbying. In 2006, nearly $100 million were spent on lobbying members of congress around issues for healthcare. Lobbying by Political Action Committees (PACs) relevant to pharmaceutical products and healthcare greatly increased between 1990 and 2006 (see Fig. 11.1). Further individual contributions also increased. Although the money goes more to Republicans than to Democrats, substantial contributions from health-related PACs go to both parties. Much of the effort is to gain reimbursement for services offered in the Medicare or Medicaid programs. In these programs, services are likely to be reimbursed if they are included in guidelines.

Conflict of interest is another important problem that requires attention. Choudhry and a group of colleagues in Toronto surveyed contributors to clinical practice guidelines in North America. They found that 87 percent of the guideline authors had some form of interaction with an industry that made a product relevant to the guidelines they were creating and 58 percent had received direct financial support from these industries. On an average, the authors of the guidelines had interacted with 10 different companies [11]. Another study obtained disclosures from 685 contributors to medical guideline committees. It found that more than a third of the statements revealed conflicts of interest [12]. There are many other examples of these conflicts. In fact, most investigators who have taken the time to look for conflicts have found them. One of the most notable cases was the development of the National Cholesterol

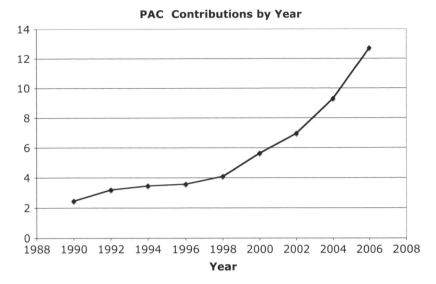

Fig. 11.1 Money spent by Political Action Committees on health pharmaceutical lobbying between 1990 and 2006. (Data from Center for Responsible Politics).

Education Program. In 2004, new guidelines for cholesterol management were developed (see Chapter 7). When the guidelines were first published by the National Heart, Lung, and Blood Institute, the American Heart Association, and the American College of Cardiology, the article did not include conflict of interest disclosures. An editorial in the "New York Times" raised the concern. So, the organizations produced the disclosures on their websites. What was revealed was that most of the committee members did, indeed, have cozy financial entanglements with the manufacturers of statin drugs—precisely the medications that the guidelines promoted. There is clearly a need for disclosure or something stronger [13].

In 2007, the US Food and Drug Administration proposed stricter disclosures for its panel members, including a requirement of full disclosure of financial relationships between FDA advisors and commercial interests at least 30 days before a meeting. Reaction to the proposal was described as "lukewarm" [14]. Creating a stricter system will be a challenge, but it will be worth it.

Disclosure may be helpful, but disclosure alone will not resolve the problems. Other groups have gone further to assure independence between guideline developers and commercial entities. Medical research is an expensive enterprise and controlling conflicts of interest is challenging. A growing portion of medical research is now done outside of academic institutions and industry has become the leading funder of biomedical research. Industry also provides much of the funding for evidence-based reviews and practice guideline development.

These guidelines determine what services are delivered to patients and how doctors are evaluated. We must face the moral dilemma created by wealthy companies supporting guidelines that expand the markets for their products.

The best way to achieve independence between companies and guidelines is to create an impartial public agency to oversee guideline development. The UK already has the National Institute for Health and Clinical Excellence (NICE) that is effectively achieving this task. NICE is an independent organization that has developed clinical guidance on a significant number of healthcare topics. Participants on NICE panels are required to sign a confidentiality form, agree to a code of conduct, and declare conflicts of interest. The budget for NICE is about $50 million per year. Although this sounds expensive, it is a small fraction of what is spent on the unnecessary medical care that proper guidelines can eliminate. Of course, NICE is not immune from political pressure. Pfizer, for example, asked the British court to block a NICE recommendation that restricted the use of their drug for Alzheimer's disease [15]. Nevertheless, NICE has done an excellent job of providing distance between themselves and companies that apply political pressure.

The Institute of Medicine of the National Academies of Science is currently developing guidelines and other tools that can be used to manage conflicts of interest without harming constructive collaboration between the public and the private sectors. Their report and guidance should be publicly available soon.

- Evidence-based guidelines should be required to consider both costs and opportunity costs.

We need to get value for the money we spend on healthcare. Not all treatments afford an equal level of benefit to patients. Some offer only minor benefits, while others produce substantial changes in patient outcome. Furthermore, the costs to produce a unit of benefit differ dramatically across treatment options. Until recently, healthcare decision-makers expressed little interest in estimating value for patients. But with shrinking budgets and an every-increasing menu of attractive options, it is no longer ethical to advocate for every option. We must concentrate on choices that offer the best value for the communities served. Quality healthcare is what makes patients better. Quality healthcare management uses resources to improve the health of populations and not spend money to purchase services that are unlikely to extend life or improve life quality.

There is substantial variability in the use of healthcare services in different countries and in different communities within countries. Healthcare providers often order tests and provide treatments that have limited value for patients. Excessive healthcare utilization increases the cost of healthcare without necessarily producing benefits. Aggressive approaches to diagnoses and treatment result in overestimates of illness within communities. Many people are diagnosed with health problems, and substantial proportions of all populations consume prescription medications. Often, these treatments result in better patient outcomes. However, the inflation of illness through overdiagnosis also leads to the inappropriate use of resources, high costs, and exposure of patients to medical errors and potentially harmful side effects of treatment.

Advocates in healthcare often argue that their programs require more resources. Cardiologists argue that more tests and procedures should be funded. Oncologists press for greater use of screening, chemotherapy, and new approaches to tumor management. Pediatricians argue that more money must be spent on children. All of the specialties argue for something similar. They need more money.

Although economists study costs, they define costs very broadly. Most people think of costs only in terms of money. Accountants consider how much money must be devoted to each alternative. Economists use the term "cost" in a broader sense. For them, a cost is what must be surrendered to obtain a particular alternative. For example, recovery from surgery is a cost of the choice to have an operation. A hospital's investment in a cancer-screening program might mean that there are not enough resources to purchase new operating-room equipment. Costs describe what is traded off when a decision is made. Some costs are monetary, and some costs reflect nonmonetary trade-offs. Monetary costs are relatively easy to quantify. Some of the other costs require new assessment methodologies.

Chapter 9 reviewed cost-effectiveness methods that are gaining increasing attention in health care. For example, by defining a common unit of health benefit, such as the QALY, it is possible to make broad comparisons between programs that may have very different specific objectives. Cost/QALY analysis permits the comparison of alternatives as different as smoking prevention for teenagers with rescue lung surgery for older adults. Some people believe that cost-effectiveness analysis is a pathway to cutting costs. The purpose of cost-effectiveness analysis is not to save money, but instead to gain value for money. In fact, most advocates for these methods would prefer to keep budgets constant or to increase them. The purpose of cost-effectiveness analysis is to save lives, not to save money. Thoughtful analysis can be used to gain the greatest value for the resources available to decision-makers.

The resistance to requiring cost-effectiveness as a component of guideline development is ill founded. It is based on the incorrect belief that the sole purpose of the analysis is to cut costs. At the end of the day, we must make choices and thoughtful analysis can guide us in the right direction.

We must also recognize that healthcare is part of a larger system. Resources used for healthcare could be used for other purposes. Decisions are complicated, and using resources for one opportunity often has the unintended consequence of limiting opportunities to support other worthy programs.

Disease, diagnosis, and dollars are all connected. Accurate and early diagnoses may combat disease and in many cases drugs save lives. However, there are other cases in which diagnosis and treatment have relatively little effect on disease, and the recommendation for using them has more to do with money than it does to the relief of human suffering. When too many dollars are used in pursuit of treatments without value, less is available to purchase services that are truly necessary. Solutions to our problems in healthcare will be difficult, but they are not impossible. Our goal is to make populations healthy, and we need to direct our resources to achieve that goal.

References

1. Anderson GF, Hussey PS, Frogner BK, Waters HR. Health spending in the United States and the rest of the industrialized world. *Health Aff (Millwood)*. 2005;245:903–914.
2. Smith C, Cowan C, Heffler S, Catlin A. National health spending in 2004: recent slow-down led by prescription drug spending. *Health Aff (Millwood)*. 2006;255:186–196.
3. Emanuel EJ, Fuchs VR. Who really pays for health care? The myth of "shared responsibility". *JAMA*. 2008;2995:1057–1059.
4. Golomb B, Evans M. Risk factors for rhabdomyolysis with simvastatin and atorvastatin. *Drug Saf*. 2006;295:1191; author reply – 2.
5. Lepkifker E, Sverdlik A, Iancu I, Ziv R, Segev S, Kotler M. Renal insufficiency in long-term lithium treatment. *J Clin Psychiatry*. 2004;655:850–856.
6. Shah NS, Wright A, Bai GH, et al. Worldwide emergence of extensively drug-resistant tuberculosis. *Emerg Infect Dis*. 2007;135:380–387.
7. Zhang J, Ding EL, Song Y. Adverse effects of cyclooxygenase 2 inhibitors on renal and arrhythmia events: meta-analysis of randomized trials. *JAMA*. 2006;2965:1619–32.
8. Bhatnagar V, Stewart ST, Huynh V, Jorgensen G, Kaplan RM. Estimating the risk of long-term erectile, urinary and bowel symptoms resulting from prostate cancer treatment. *Prostate Cancer Prostatic Dis*. 2006;95:136–146.
9. Gellad ZF, Lyles KW. Direct-to-consumer advertising of pharmaceuticals. *Am J Med*. 2007;1205:475–480.
10. Frosch DL, Krueger PM, Hornik RC, Cronholm PF, Barg FK. Creating demand for prescription drugs: a content analysis of television direct-to-consumer advertising. *Ann Fam Med*. 2007;55:6–13.
11. Choudhry NK, Stelfox HT, Detsky AS. Relationships between authors of clinical practice guidelines and the pharmaceutical industry. *Am Med Assoc*. 2002;2875:612–617.
12. Hasenfeld R, Shekelle PG. Is the methodological quality of guidelines declining in the US? Comparison of the quality of US Agency for Health Care Policy and Research (AHCPR) guidelines with those published subsequently. *Qual Saf Health Care*. 2003;125:428–434.
13. Steinbrook R. Guidance for guidelines. *N Engl J Med*. 2007;3565:331–333.
14. Finkelstein JB. Proposed FDA conflict-of-interest guidelines get lukewarm reception. *J Natl Cancer Inst*. 2007;995:747–788.
15. Steinbrook R. Guidance for guidelines. *N Engl J Med*. 2007;3565:331–333.

Index

Printed in the United States of America